G000061288

Dentist on the Ward

2016 (6ᵗʰ) Edition

An Introduction to Oral and Maxillofacial Surgery for Postgraduate Core Trainees in Dentistry

Andrew Sadler and Leo Cheng

Dentist on the Ward

Copyright © Andrew Sadler 2016

www.dentist-on-the-ward.co.uk

All Rights Reserved

No part of this book may be reproduced, stored in a retrieval system, or transmitted, in any form or by any means, electronic, mechanical, photocopying, recording or otherwise without prior permission of the copyright owner. The Authors assert their moral right to be identified as the authors of this work.

First Edition Published   2010

2011-12 Edition Published 2011

Third Edition 2013

Fourth Edition 2014

2015 (5th) Edition 2015

2016 (6th) Edition 2016

ISBN: 978-0-9569377-5-9

Dentist on the Ward

www.dentist-on-the-ward.co.uk

©Andrew Sadler 2016

Preface to 6th Edition

This text is written for students and recently qualified dental surgeons working in hospital departments of Oral and Maxillofacial Surgery for the first time. It arose from our 'Dentist on the Ward' courses started in Lincoln in 1995.

Like the course the text is intended as an introduction for those with no prior experience.

The text includes information broadly in four categories:-

1. An introduction to the hospital and essential information necessary for the new recruit who is not medically qualified.

2. Advice on routine procedures which the new appointee may have to carry out on their own.

3. Background clinical information which relates to these procedures and includes much basic knowledge on medical subjects relevant to oral surgery or dentistry.

4. An introduction to the clinical work of Oral & Maxillofacial Surgeons as practised in the United Kingdom designed to help understanding of the work. These chapters have the words 'Introduction' or 'Understanding' in their titles. These chapters are intended to be succinct for easy reading in a short time but we believe they cover the essential elements required for examination candidates at undergraduate and general postgraduate general examinations in dentistry but not specialist examinations.

The book is edited, expanded and updated with a new edition each year to take account of changes in practice, regulation and hospital procedures.

For the 6th edition eight chapters have been updated to include changes in clinical practice; four new chapters have been added and two old ones removed.

The text is copyright and may not be copied in part or whole.

Andrew Sadler and Leo Cheng. January 2016

Acknowledgements

Oral and Maxillofacial Surgery as well as hospital medicine and nursing have become more complicated and specialised so in spite of the fact that this book is aimed at basic post graduate trainees it becomes more difficult to keep up to date in every aspect of the subjects we have written about. We have therefore become more reliant on advice and help from friends and colleagues.

We would like to acknowledge the help of the following who have read our initial texts and pointed out errors and omissions and suggested changes of emphasis. These are Richard Thornton (Consultant Anaesthetist), Nayeem Ali and Martin Clark (Consultant OMFS Surgeons), Tom Sheehan (Consultant Oncologist). In addition help in other ways was given by Rob Scott (Consultant Anaesthetist), Malcolm Read (Consultant Head & Neck Pathologist), Graham Griffiths (Consultant Chemical Pathologist), Elaine Purbrick & Amanda Syson (Registered General Nurses).

Table of Contents

1. <u>Why work in Oral and Maxillofacial Surgery</u>?

The speciality of Oral and Maxillofacial Surgery (OMFS) has evolved within the National Health Service from old hospital dental departments (whose work was mostly tooth removal) and a few 'Departments of Jaw Injuries' which were formed to deal with war injuries under the charge of Plastic Surgeons.

Nowadays, much of the time of the Consultants in OMFS will be taken up with the management of cancer, trauma, facial deformity and salivary gland disease which 40 years ago were likely to have been managed by other specialties. However, despite this and long overdue initiatives by the purchasers of NHS care in the UK to move Minor Oral Surgery away from hospitals and into specialist practices, the majority of work coming into departments of OMFS is of direct relevance to dentistry. This work provides a wealth of potential learning material for the recently qualified dental surgeon; this includes oral medicine, temporomandibular joint problems, facial pain as well as dento-alveolar surgery and extraction work on the medically compromised.

Dental Core Training (Year 1) posts in OMFS are mostly re-badged Senior House Officer (SHO) jobs. In addition there are a number of Dental Core Training Year 2 and 3, 'Career Development' and 'Clinical Fellowships' funded by individual hospital trusts available to dental surgeons at the beginning of their careers. These jobs will give valuable experience in the speciality and core generic skills transferable to other branches of dentistry.

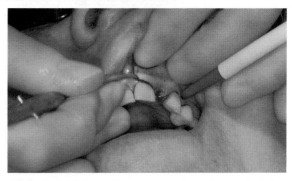

You should be able to treat most dento-alveolar conditions.

The most beneficial time to take a junior post in OMFS is soon after qualifying following on from the Vocational Training (Foundation Year) in dental practice. At this time you will have developed some considerable skill in the handling of anxious patients, some considerable dexterity in carrying out operative procedures, and an understanding of dentistry within the primary care sector; this will be of help in understanding the problems of those who refer patients

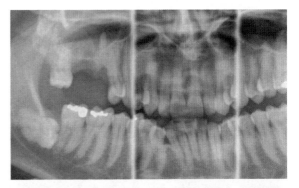

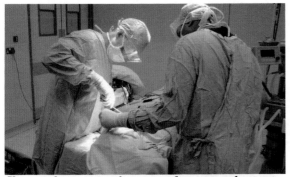

You can learn to work as part of a team and operate on simple trauma and dento-alveolar conditions as well as assisting in major cases.

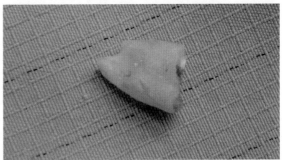

You will learn the management of complications such as this root displaced into the maxillary antrum.

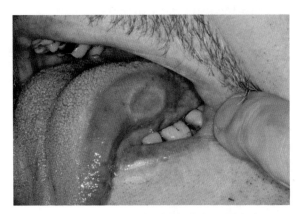

You should see lots of Oral Medicine. This is not a cancer but a Nicorandil ulcer on the tongue.

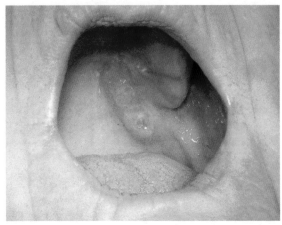

The significance of this lymphoma on the palate was missed by the dentist who eased the patient's denture away from it. An OMFS department is the best place to become familiar with dangerous oral conditions.

into the Hospital. You may be able to pass on some of this benefit to your senior colleagues who have not worked in primary care dentistry for many years, if at all.

The main reason to take a job will remain the opportunity to learn but you can also expect it to be fun. It may be the first time that you are working as part of a team managing individual patients. Team working can be enjoyable, especially in times of difficulty, and the camaraderie and sense of common purpose gives added enjoyment to the work. It is probable that, at least at the beginning, you will discuss almost every patient you see with another colleague, which is unlikely to be the case in dental practice.

Most jobs you apply for will be for six months or one year, or if they are in a dental teaching hospital they may rotate through other specialist departments of dentistry. At the end of this time we would usually recommend moving on rather than staying longer in the same department. If you are intending to work elsewhere within dentistry you have probably got as much out of the speciality as you are going to and if you intend to have a career in OMFS then it will probably be better in the long term to complement your experience elsewhere as a dental core trainee year 2, or in a career development or clinical fellow post.

In practical terms, at the end of a one year post you should aim to be competent at performing most dental extractions (surgical or otherwise), the initial management of dental trauma, interpretation of dental radiographs and some facial X-rays and CT scans. You should have seen most common oral mucosal conditions, some maxillofacial prosthetics and implantology, patients with chronic facial pain and

some orthognathic surgery. In some units you may have seen patients with cleft lip and palate and other developmental anomalies. You will hopefully have an understanding of temporo-mandibular joint disorders, outpatient management of patients with common co-existing medical problems, working relationships with other disciplines such as orthodontics, restorative dentistry and ENT surgery and the issues regarding general anaesthesia and conscious sedation. You should also understand clinical governance and have participated in clinical audit. The best way to study for postgraduate examinations is to read around and discuss clinical cases and you should have seen plenty of clinical material to help you with either the Royal College of Surgeons of England MJDF or Royal College of Surgeons of Edinburgh MFDS examinations.

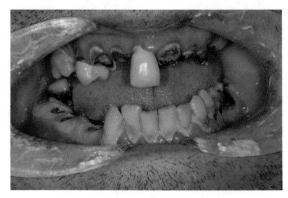

You should be able to carry out a lot of surgical extractions.

2. Applying for a job in Oral and Maxillofacial Surgery

For many recently qualified dental surgeons access to OMFS training will be as a Dental Core Trainee year 1, (formerly called Foundation Training Year 2 or Senior House Officer). There will usually be centralized application with a process of matching candidates to jobs; a long application form must be completed and will be 'scored' by an assessor. Candidates will be ranked in order of desirability by their ability to fill in a form rather than potential to benefit from training.

The first decision to make is where to apply. This may to a certain extent be decided by what your future career intentions may be. If you think that you may wish to pursue a career in the speciality you will need to study Medicine and it would be advantageous to work in a department which can demonstrate a well-trodden path from OMFS house job to medical student. This may well be in the OMFS unit in the teaching hospital from where you qualified; it may also be in a high profile unit in a hospital with a medical school but no dental hospital. Make sure you do your homework and find out what the record of placing dentally qualified house surgeons in the medical school is.

It is most important that you find out about the departments in which you might work as you are going to invest six months or a year of your life there. There are still many units which provide inferior jobs for their junior trainees, or where it may simply be not very pleasant to work. If you can, try to work in a single site unit. Avoid jobs where you will be expected to drive between different hospitals at night to sew up drunks, or where you might have to work in a hospital peripheral to the main unit at a time when there is no one senior present to advise or help you. Be wary of jobs where there are many house surgeons working shifts to cover busy trauma commitments at night. If you are going to be working a night shift, working time regulations mean you will not be able to work during the day which is when the minor oral surgery and oral medicine cases that you will need to see for your training will be attending.

Check that there is sufficient clinical work in the department for the number of house surgeons and that when carrying out minor oral surgery there is adequate support, supervision and teaching. You can do this by

> ### Typical questions on centralised application form for Dental Core Training (Yr .1) application form
>
> 1. Describe how the Vocational Training experience has improved your care of patients
>
> 2. Give two examples from clinical dentistry where you have felt less competent & what steps you have taken to address this
>
> 3. List five reasons you want to be a Core Trainee
>
> 4. Describe any management duties you have undertaken. How has the experience been of benefit?

speaking to the present incumbents. Always ask direct questions and talk to more than one to get a balanced picture; be wary of over enthusiastic reports as some young people can be uncritical and sycophantic to their seniors beyond justification. Give an especially wide berth to departments where the trainees run errands or get little supervised operating experience. You may possibly find that practical surgical experience is given preferentially to second or third year dental core trainees and those in the first year get little or none. This will most likely be that in order to cover the on-call rotas and remain compliant with European working time regulations there are too many trainees for the supervised surgical training available. If this is the situation you may want to walk away and apply to a smaller unit - we would. Practical operating experience is the foundation of learning surgery.

All NHS Trusts have to abide by current employment law with regard to appointments and this will cover discrimination on grounds of sex, race (colour, nationality, ethnic or national origins), marital status, religion, sexual orientation, disability and age. In order that there may be no accusations on any of these grounds after a post has been appointed, they are all advertised nationally. Most jobs now will be advertised by the schools of postgraduate dentistry in the British Dental Journal but you should also keep an eye on www.jobs.nhs.uk.

All advertised posts should have a job description which should contain an accurate description of the duties, rotas and timetable. These will subsequently form part of the contract of employment. Most importantly amongst the documents will be a 'Personal Specification' which is a list of essential and desirable requirements of the successful applicants. This list is important as it will be used as the bench mark as to whom is to be shortlisted.

Always complete all parts of the application. If not completed it may be assumed that the candidate is omitting something which will cast an unfavourable light on them. Many applications now will be on-line rather than paper and you may not be able to submit a CV.

When filling in the application pay close attention to the job description and personal specification and match your answers to that. It will be useful if you have thought of, and preferably committed to writing, a personal development plan. This should include what your immediate learning and training objectives are. Try to match the experience in the job applied for to your training needs as in your personal development plan. Do not feel obliged to state what your long term career objectives are if you have not yet decided.

If you are allowed to submit a printed CV keep it short, certainly no more than two sides of A4; to make it longer risks it not being read. Keep it neat, printed on one side and fastened with only one staple at the corner and no fancy binders which will have to be removed for photocopying. The expense and trouble of using heavy expensive paper will be wasted as it will be a photocopy that is seen by the selection committee.

If you have won prizes at school or undergraduate level you can list them in your application or CV; it may be that someone will be impressed. Lastly, you should give the names of two referees, one of whom should be from your most recent employment. The Human Resources Department will require a reference to be on record for all staff but it is almost certain that what is said in the reference will have little bearing whether a person is appointed, unless it is very bad. Not using a referee from your present or most recent employment will usually be considered with suspicion.

The most important aspect of the whole application procedure is not to lie or confabulate. You will be surprised how often this occurs and is most common on the subject of publications and career intentions. If you say on your application that you have submitted a paper for publication be prepared to be asked about it at interview; otherwise leave it out. If you are found

---

> **Some typical essential criteria for Dental Core Training (Yr. 1) application**
>
> 1. Registration with GDC
> 2. BDS (or equivalent)
> 3. Satisfactory completion of VT
> 4. Not more than 30 months post-grad experience
> 5. Basic life support skills
> 6. Awareness of own limitations
> 7. Understand clinical risk management
> 8. Competent to work without direct supervision where appropriate
> 9. Good manual dexterity and hand/eye co-ordination
> 10. Appropriate clinical knowledge
> 11. Ability to prioritise clinical need
> 12. Ability to organise oneself and own work
> 13. Experience and ability to work in multi-professional teams
> 14. Understand NHS clinical governance & resource constraints

---

out attempting to mislead by omitting that your paper has been submitted but rejected or if questioning reveals you don't know much about it then don't be surprised if your application fails.

The normal procedure is that everyone who submits an application and whose qualities fulfil the essential criteria on the personal specification will be considered to be shortlisted. However this may mean that there are too many candidates for interview. In these circumstances the person responsible for short listing will then move on to the desirable criteria and pick out only those who have fulfilled these. If you do not meet any of these do not be too alarmed as they will inevitably vary between individual postgraduate dental schools or departments and you will probably be considered a very desirable candidate elsewhere.

We would counsel against telephoning and asking for an appointment to see the Consultants after the job has been advertised. For a Consultant appointment it would be unusual for a serious candidate not to turn up to show and express their interest prior to interview but at Core Trainee level this is more likely to be regarded as a nuisance. We think it is far more useful to speak to one or more of the trainees in post, perhaps during an evening or week-end when they are less busy. Most will be very happy to give you all the information that you will need to decide if you wish to proceed with the application, and the information that you have visited will almost certainly be passed to the Consultants. However, it is not worthwhile your making the effort unless you know you have been shortlisted.

If you are selected for interview, turn up looking relaxed, smart and on time. Answer the questions truthfully. It is wise to prepare some answers to questions that might be anticipated, such as why you want this job, what your career intentions might be, etc. Try to look objectively at your application and CV and talk about the things you have done. At the end of the interview you may be asked if you have any questions. In our experience most candidates at this level feel they are required to ask a question, but this can be where an apparently strong candidate can make

a fool of himself or herself. In many cases now there will be many candidates being interviewed simultaneously. The selectors will give scores to each of the candidates over a number of domains. At the end the final scores are ranked and matched with the choices they have made; those who score the highest will get the better choice from the jobs available.

Suggested format for CV.

CURRICULUM VITAE:	Rob Undergreen
Name:	Robert Andrew Undergreen
Contact address:	Flat 12, Westwood House 2 Greetback Road Lincoln, LN87AZ
Telephone:	01522 897168 (H) 07968 387592 (M)
E-mail:	UnderRob@1874yahoo.com
Date of birth:	30.08.1989
Place of birth:	Skipton Yorkshire
Nationality:	British
GDC Registration:	Full No: 80271
Present Appt.:	General Dental Practice. Locum From August 2005 to date. Braces Dental Practice, Cobham Surrey.
Previous Appt.:	Vocational Trainee From August 2004 to July 2005 Broadgate Dental Surgery, Lincoln

Education:	University of Nottingham Dental School 2004 - 2009 BDS.
	Woodhall Spa High School 1998- 2004 A levels Chemistry, Physics and Drama.
Awards:	Horncastle Sports Club. 100 metres winner 2003 .
Elective Study:	Attachment to Periodontology Department: Bangalore General Hospital India 2007. Undergraduate elective.
Hobbies:	Creative writing. Photography.
Career Aim:	I wish to gain experience and confidence in Oral Surgery & Oral Medicine and pass the MJDF. I wish to specialise in a branch of clinical dentistry.
Referees :	Mr Stephen Whiterock, Broadgate Dental Surgery, East Parade, Lincoln LN8 8PF
	Professor T R Tranthumh University Dental School of Nottingham, Nottingham NG16 8YR

3. <u>Getting the Best from a Student Elective</u>

Several universities arrange for their dental students to have attachments to OMFS departments. We believe that the experience gained from such an attachment will be enhanced by a little thought and planning before starting and a proactive attitude on arrival. Our experience is that Consultants are generally keen to have students in their departments and Specialist Registrars and Core Trainees are often very willing to go out of their way to help and teach them.

Our advice is to go with a 'shopping list' of types of clinical cases you wish to see. Take a history from the patients (ask if you can), examine them, look up what investigations have been done, see the results, ask questions and read around the cases. Ideally you should present the cases to someone such as a Consultant or Specialist Registrar and provoke a discussion on the management of the patient from which you can learn. It is best to choose cases which will be of use to you in preparation for your examinations or practice of dentistry.

You should ask if you can attend the operating theatre if minor oral surgery is being carried out under anaesthetic or sedation, and assist the surgeon. If you are lucky you may be allowed to carry out some practical procedures such as exodontia. When in theatre ask the anaesthetist if he or she will teach you venepuncture as this is a useful skill you may need later if carrying out sedation. Above all, make sure you see and palpate any new mouth cancers presenting to the department during your attachment and find out the history from the patient. Try to avoid spending long hours in the theatre watching long cancer cases unless you are able to get some practice at suturing.

If you wish to undertake a longer elective write some time in advance. In these circumstances it is usual to undertake a small research or audit project. Visit the hospital a few months beforehand for a discussion with a Consultant who may have some pet topics or projects which may interest you for study in greater depth.

List of priority things to do on student elective

1. Hands on practice at exodontia & minor oral surgery if possible, particularly if there are dental extractions under general anaesthetic

2. See patients presenting with oral cancer. Listen to the history, examine & palpate the lesion & lymphatic drainage, follow the investigation & find out what the treatment is to be

3. Get experience in venepuncture; particularly ask the anaesthetist to teach you in theatre

4. Take a full history from a patient with an oral medical condition, see several with white patches in the mouth & learn which ones might be precancerous & which ones you would refer in if you were working in dental practice

5. Take a history from a patient with post extraction haemorrhage, note their management & what tests and observations are done & why. See a patient with post extraction osteitis

6. Take a history and examine a patient with a severe dental abscess; note their investigation and management

7. See a patient with a fractured mandible, particularly observe the management of dental injuries & use this as a basis for learning current management of dental trauma

8. Observe hospital cross infection control

9. Attend a clinical governance meeting

10. See some orthognathic surgery; you must see the patient before and after the surgery to appreciate the problem. (Do this for all patients whose surgery you observe if possible.)

11. See a major cancer operation but don't waste all day observing one case unless you get some suturing practice

4. <u>Education, Personal Development and Appraisal</u>

The whole purpose of the job, from your point of view, is to enhance your postgraduate education. If, before you start, you are unsure how your personal and clinical skills might develop during the year, you should reflect on it within the first few weeks and come up with your ideas. Initially most young dentists will be primarily concerned with finding their way around their duties and settling in. Afterwards come concerns about whether they are going to cope without disappointing their seniors; this is natural and usual. Once you have settled in do try to formulate what you want to get out of the job and voice this at your first appraisal.

Ideally the job should provide you with a wealth of clinical material (patients) whose treatment you can observe and participate in with sufficient supervision that you can learn. Initially you should expect supervision to be very close and later more relaxed but within a framework of guidance you have received. There should be clinical meetings:- journal discussions, clinico-pathological conferences, clinical governance and morbidity and mortality meetings where cases are discussed. There should always be someone available when you are treating patients to give help or guidance and occasionally take over if you are having difficulty.

During the post you should have a named educational supervisor who should act as a mentor, provide guidance in your learning, give you feedback about your performance and, if necessary, provide pastoral support. The educational supervisor will normally be one of the Consultants you work with. This relationship may be formalised by you both signing an 'Educational Contract'. They may provide feedback to the director of the training programme and the postgraduate dental dean. The main frame work of this relationship should be appraisal meetings which normally take place soon after the start, at six months and near the end of your year. These are not assessments but should be an opportunity for feedback of performance and for you to give feedback on the value and shortcomings of the training you are receiving.

At the first appraisal you should discuss your Personal Development Plan. This should be a short list of the goals you wish to achieve. Our experience

---

> **_Example of Topics to Discuss at first Appraisal_**
>
> 1. Previous experience in last job
>
> 2. Accommodation arrangements
>
> 3. Problems encountered so far
>
> 4. Thoughts on future career
>
> 5. Aspirations for the job
>
> 6. Audit project
>
> 7. Postgraduate examinations
>
> 8 Areas of special interest or need

---

has been that the most popular and possibly the most useful goal is practical experience in minor oral surgery. In this respect it is useful to keep a log of the number of cases you have performed and assisted at. This is useful in assessing whether you are getting sufficient practical experience, and for the educational supervisor to feed back to his colleagues to ensure you get more if your numbers are low.

During your appointment you should keep a 'portfolio'. This will normally be in electronic form (e-portfolio). In this you should keep a record of work-based assessments you have done, multi-source feedback, a log of your activity, clinical audit you have carried out and progress in examinations. You should keep records of all training events you have attended within your place of work and elsewhere and your reflections of any benefit gained. The multi-source feedback will be obtained from your professional colleagues, complementary professionals and patients whose treatment you have participated in. The portfolio can be used as evidence when applying for future jobs and for revalidation when it is introduced in the future by the General Dental Council.

You should aim to complete one work based assessment per month. These should be carried out on a one to one basis with one of your trainers. They may take the form of observation of a clinical encounter (such as examining a trauma case or carrying out a surgical procedure), a case based discussion in which you present a case in which you have been involved or feedback on your performance from a variety of colleagues. The benefit of these is that it should give you an opportunity to reflect on your performance and gain insight in how your skills are improving or need to be improved. You should get feedback from your trainer so that you both can assess where you need further experience and help in achieving your training goals that you have defined in your personal development plan.

You should have one to one feedback from this. It will help you maintain steady progress towards your goals, help your progression in clinical ability and develop insight into where you need to make more progress. You should also participate in case-based discussions; learning is always easier if it is based on real clinical cases and you should learn to present cases to your colleagues in a clear and concise way - a skill that will remain with you for all your career.

We would recommend that you use the clinical material to prepare yourself for the examinations of one of the Colleges of Surgeons. You can choose either the membership of the Faculty of Dentistry of one of the Scottish Colleges or the Membership of the Joint Dental Faculties of the College of Surgeons of England.

You should base your learning goals on 'A Curriculum for UK Dental Foundation Training' published by the Department of Health on behalf of the Committee of Postgraduate Dental Deans and Directors and endorsed by the Faculties of Dentistry of the Surgical Royal Colleges. The best way to study is to use clinical cases to base your learning on rather than to wade through textbooks. Observe and participate in clinical practice in the Hospital, follow through individual cases, ask questions as to why things are being done, and read around them. This makes learning memorable, relevant and enjoyable.

Example of Personal Development Plan

1. Gain more confidence in diagnosis and management of white patches in the mouth

2. Remove more impacted third molars. Target : 20 cases by April

3. Finish audit project by May

4. Pass Part 2 MJDF June

The goals should follow the principle of SMART: Specific, Measurable, Achievable, Realistic and Timed.

In addition to improving your clinical skills you should also consider other skills which may be useful in your subsequent career, such as presenting cases, writing, improving your skills in the use of software and, if the opportunity arises, by helping teach dental and nursing students.

Your employing NHS Trust will insist that you receive some statutory (required by law) and mandatory (required by employer) training in various core topics. The NHS Trust will receive intermittent inspections from the Care Quality Commission and the NHS Litigation Authority and will be required to prove that its staff have received training in these topics. Mandatory training may take many forms including reading set texts and confirming in writing that you have read them, following on-line learning programmes on the Trust intranet and attendance at specific training sessions during working hours. Remember to keep records of all meetings, training and certificates in your portfolio.

Statutory and Mandatory Training topics

1. Conflict Resolution

2. Equality and Diversity

3. Fire Safety

4. Health and Safety

5. Incidents, Complaints and Claims

6. Infection Prevention and Control

7. Information Governance

8. Safeguarding Adults

9. Safeguarding Children

5. <u>Information, Data Protection and Confidentiality</u>

These topics are collectively referred to as information governance. They will form one module of the mandatory training that you will receive in post but it will be useful for you to have an idea of some of the principles and knowledge of a few not-to-dos from day one.

You will already be aware that patients have an absolute right to complete confidentiality about their condition and treatment. This extends to you having to be careful about discussing patients with colleagues where you can be overheard, leaving notes or documents in places where they may be seen by someone not involved in their care, discarding anything written about a patient in non-secure rubbish, communicating about patients by email other than by the secure NHS.net system or discussing patients out of the work environment. This right of confidentiality extends not only to the ordinary patient but anyone who is well known or famous that you have dealings with. Do not gossip.

You will probably be called upon to discuss management with relatives of patients. Relatives do not have a right to know so you must ensure that the patient consents to this, which in nearly all cases they do. However, in the few cases where patients have concerns about confidentiality it is from relatives that they often want information to be specifically withheld.

Information that you record about patients must be accurate; this will mostly be written notes. They should be legible and each note should be dated and, for inpatients, timed. The notes should be written at the time the patient is seen or an event occurs. If something is forgotten and a note is written about an event from a previous time it should be made clear in the notes when it was written.

All organisations that keep and process personal information must conform to the Data Protection Act 1998 and be registered with the Office of the Information Commissioner. The registered organisation or individual will be a 'Data Controller' and will have to register what information is kept; it must be kept secure and only the minimum information is held. This means that you cannot keep any information yourself out of your employer's premises or systems. To do so would make you a data controller for which you will not be registered, and is thus illegal.

If clinical photographs are taken of patients you should be aware of your employer's photograph policy. Clinical photographs should be available as part of a patient's record and must be stored on the hospital's computer system. Most will completely forbid pictures to be taken on mobile phones and may forbid images being made on cameras other than those belonging to the hospital trust. Images made of patients (with their consent) may be shown at clinical meetings without specific consent to do so from the patient as long as they are not identifiable. If they are identifiable then consent must be obtained. If an image (including x-rays or scans) is published then the patient must consent whether they can be identified or not. Publication means by any mode, so if you give a lecture with projection of clinical images you must not allow your presentation to be copied, emailed or deposited on a university system unless every patient has consented to this.

Any electronic patient data that you carry must be encrypted. Your employer may issue you with an encrypted memory stick for this purpose.

You should never access confidential information about patients that you have no legitimate clinical reason to do so. For example you should not access clinical investigation results for friends or relatives or anyone whose care you are not involved with.

In your first week you will probably have some training on the use of the Trust's computer system. You should ensure that you change your password as required and that you never allow anyone else to know your password. You must log off the computer system as soon as you have finished; otherwise you might allow unauthorised access to clinical records or another staff member might misuse the system and you would get blamed; its use will be monitored.

You will be aware that patients have a right to access their health records. You should always write records in the knowledge that this might occur. If a patient asks to see records or requires information that they are entitled to under the Freedom of Information Act you should inform the Trust information governance team as there will be set procedures to follow and records that will need to be made.

6. Pre-employment Health Assessment and the Blood Borne Viruses

Any offer of a job will be made to you conditionally pending the successful completion of pre-employment checks. This will include an occupational health check. You will not be asked about any health issues you may have before this conditional offer but afterwards you will be asked if you are aware of any health problem or disability which might affect your ability to perform the job.

Working in a hospital in any clinical activity presents innumerable opportunities to spread infectious agents from clinician to patient, from patient to clinician and from one patient to another. The process of reducing the risk starts with the pre-employment health screening.

Because your job will involve contact with patients and their bodily fluids you will have to undergo a 'Work Health Assessment' which will include a communicable disease questionnaire and screening. This is normally carried out by an occupational health nurse who will refer you to the occupational health physician if a problem is identified. This will normally take place as soon as you start work; you will not be allowed to carry out any 'exposure prone procedures' (see below) until you have been 'cleared'.

Among them you will be asked if you have ever worked abroad and there will be specific questions about whether you have been immunised against diphtheria, tetanus, polio, rubella, mumps, measles, influenza, varicella and Hepatitis B. If you have lived all your life and been trained in the UK this will be easy.

Hepatitis B has a low prevalence in the UK but health care workers are considered to be at higher risk and it will therefore be necessary for you to have been immunised with treated hepatitis B surface antigen (HBsAg). Normally you will already have been immunised with three doses of vaccine and tested for antibody response between 2 and 4 weeks after the final dose. The desired response is an anti-hepatitis B surface antigen (Anti -HBs) antibody titre of more than 100 mIU/ml. Written confirmation of the result will be required by the occupational health department. Some individuals do not respond well to the immunisation, particularly if they are over 40, obese or immunocompromised. An antibody titre of between 10

and 100 mIU/ml indicates a partial response which may be improved by a booster dose of vaccine. A non-responder with a titre of below 10 mIU/ml may have naturally acquired immunity and be HBsAg -ve and have antibody to the Hepatitis B core antigen (Anti-HBc +ve). However, non-responders may have current infection shown by being HBsAg +ve and Anti-HBs +ve. They should be tested for Hepatitis B e antigen (HBeAg). If they are found to be positive they will be infectious and will have to cease any exposure prone procedures. Hepatitis B is a Prescribed Industrial Disease for Health Care Workers, and compensation is available under the NHS Injuries Benefit Scheme.

Non-responders to the vaccination who are not HBsAg +ve can work but are at a greater risk from patients. Anyone who is HBsAg +ve but not HBeAg +ve may be able to work, depending upon their viral load which will need to be tested.

From 2003 onwards anyone new to clinical practice or starting training has had to be tested for antibodies to hepatitis C virus RNA. Carriers of Hepatitis C virus RNA are infectious and should not carry out exposure prone procedures. It is possible that anti-viral treatment may reverse this and work can be resumed if they are found to be negative for the virus six months later. There have been only a few incidents of hepatitis C infection of patients by health care workers. Anyone who has been trained in the UK will have been tested and will have been given documentary evidence; otherwise the new recruit will need to be tested and produce a driving licence or passport to verify their identity.

All health care workers in the UK, of whatever profession, have ethical obligations concerning HIV. Until recently they have not been allowed to undertake exposure prone procedures if they have a reason to suspect that they may have HIV. New health care workers are obliged to be tested and are obliged to seek advice from an occupational health department, who will test and, if positive, arrange treatment and advice. The Department of Health has modified its guidance and from April 2014 heath care workers who are HIV positive may carry out exposure prone procedures provided they are taking effective anti-retroviral drug therapy, they have an undetectable viral load and are monitored by an occupational health physician. Self-testing kits are now available for HIV.

The number of cases of tuberculosis has been increasing slowly in the UK in recent years. Hospital staff are considered to be high risk, as are patients in hospital, particularly the elderly and immunocompromised. If you have been brought up in the UK and have been to a UK dental school then you will have been immunised with Bacillus Calmette Guérin freeze dried live attenuated Mycobacterium Bovis (BCG) and should therefore be at low risk. If you are from abroad, particularly from Africa or the Indian sub-continent, you will need to have a chest X-ray. If you have not had BCG, as witnessed by the typical skin marking, you will need a Mantoux tuberculin test to determine if you have immunity. If this fails to show immunity then it will still be possible for you to start work, but you will need the BCG vaccination. If you exhibit a very strong reaction to Mantoux this may indicate that you have active disease, and further investigation and treatment may be needed.

Most adults in the UK will have had chicken pox, caused by the herpes zoster virus, in childhood when it is usually a mild illness. Your antibody status should have been checked if you have been through a UK dental school. If you are not immune, you are susceptible to catching the disease from close contact with an infected patient; it will be a more severe illness in adulthood. Should you contract chicken pox you may be infectious during the period from two days before the rash appears until the skin lesions crust over. If a woman contracts chicken pox up to the 20th week of pregnancy the foetus may be damaged. You should therefore know if you are immune or not. If you have not been previously tested for varicella antibodies this will be done. If negative you will be given two doses of vaccine 4 to 8 weeks apart.

Like chicken pox, rubella is a mild illness usually but it can be devastating to the foetus if contracted within the first ten weeks of pregnancy with 90% of foetuses having malformations, which may be multiple. Most children in the UK are protected by vaccination with the MMR (Measles, Mumps, Rubella vaccine). If you have been trained in the UK you will have had your rubella immunity checked. If not, this can be done by the occupational health department.

Exposure Prone Procedures

These are invasive procedures where there is a risk that injury may result in the exposure of the patient's open tissues to the blood of the worker. They include procedures where the worker's gloved hands may be in contact with sharp instruments, needle tips and sharp tissues (spicules of bone and teeth) inside a patient's open body cavity, wound or confined anatomical space, where the hands or finger tips may not be completely visible at all times (Department of Health 2003). This will include all clinical dentistry except complete denture prosthodontics. The taking of blood, setting up and maintaining IV lines and minor surface suturing are not exposure prone procedures as the whole of the hands are visible at all times.

7. <u>Hospital Cross Infection Control: MRSA, Clostridium Difficile and Hand Hygiene</u>

Staphylococcus aureus is common in air, clothing, bedding and dust, where it can survive for several weeks. It is also carried by approximately 40% of healthy adults in their noses and, to a lesser extent, in their throats and faeces. It can develop resistance to antibiotics by adaptation and can flourish at the expense of antibiotic sensitive organisms.

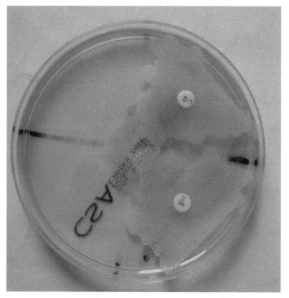

MRSA. Growth is uninhibited by the Oxycycline discs.

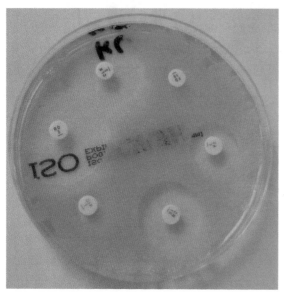

Staphylococcus aureus on agar plate. Sensitivity is indicated by the inhibition of growth by antibiotics discs.

The most commonly used antibiotic for treating Staph. aureus infection is Flucloxacillin; when the organism is resistant to Flucloxacillin it is known as MRSA (Methicillin Resistant Staphylococcus Aureus). This is because the older drug Methicillin is used to test sensitivity because in vitro it accurately mimics the in vivo behaviour of Flucloxacillin. In fact Oxycycline is commonly used for testing nowadays but it is still known as MRSA. MRSA has been known, and been increasing in prevalence, since the 1960s.

MRSA and other drug resistant bacteria exist because of over-use of antibiotics; it is therefore essential for all clinicians to use antibiotics sparingly for those few patients who really need them for serious infection. Dentists are notorious for over using antibiotics, which should never be prescribed for minor dental infections as an alternative to pulp extirpation or tooth extraction. It is nonsense to prescribe antibiotics

to reduce acute inflammation before a local anaesthetic is given.

Patients and others can be 'colonised' by MRSA without any pathogenic response. They are said to have become 'infected' when the patient develops inflammatory signs or symptoms.

The greatest risk of MRSA is in those patients who have surgical wounds, are immunocompromised or have serious debilitating illness. It is of low risk to those in outpatient clinics, paediatric or general medical wards, but the risk will be greater in the intensive care, oncology and renal wards.

The mainstay of prevention of colonisation and infection of patients with MRSA is a high standard of routine cross infection control, such as hand washing, using protective clothing, good cleaning and isolation of colonised or infected patients.

Those who are admitted to a surgical ward by transfer from a facility with a high risk of colonisation are screened by taking swabs for culture from their hairline, nostrils, axillae, groin and any wounds. This will include patients transferred from other hospitals or nursing homes. A patient found to be infected or colonised is 'barrier nursed' in a single room. The room should be maintained clean and tidy and contain no unnecessary furniture. Staff entering should wear gloves and aprons which should be disposed of on leaving the room. Staff should enter only when necessary; wounds should be covered and strict hand hygiene should be observed.

Patients colonised by MRSA may be decolonised by using Mupirocin 2% ointment to the nostrils three times a day; antiseptic detergent should be used for a total body bath or shower which should include the hair; colonised wounds should be treated with Povidone-iodine. If staff are found to be colonised then an attempt should be made to reverse this with Mupirocin. If working in high risk areas such as intensive care or the renal unit then they may have to cease work temporarily until decontaminated and have had three consecutive negative swabs from hairline, nostrils, axillae and groin.

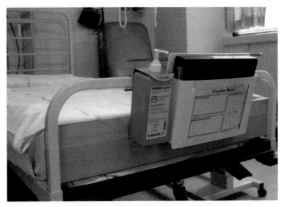

Alcoholic hand rub containers are placed strategically throughout wards and clinical areas. Here at the end of a bed for use on ward rounds.

Hand Hygiene

Good hand hygiene is probably the single most important method of combating cross infection. You will find there are many hand wash basins with soap and taps that can be controlled with elbows available in all clinical areas of the hospital. Hands should be washed before and after starting work, after using the toilet, before eating, and when the hands are obviously contaminated. In addition to this the hands must be cleaned with an alcohol rub on entering or leaving a ward or clinical area, in between seeing patients and before carrying out an aseptic procedure. Containers with alcohol rub will be available at all hand basins and at the entrance to and within all clinical areas as well at the end of beds on the wards. The alcohol rub should only be used on visibly clean hands; otherwise they should be washed with soap and water beforehand. Hand cream will also be available in ward areas and should be used after high frequency of hand washing, before breaks and at the end of work.

Clostridium difficile, commonly referred to as C. diff., is an anaerobic bacterium which lives harmlessly in the gut of approximately 3% of the normal population. It is usually kept in check by other commensal gut organisms but if these are reduced by broad spectrum antibiotics then C. diff. can propagate in large amounts, releasing Toxin A and Toxin B which can damage the gut wall leading to ulceration, bleeding and diarrhoea. The diarrhoea can vary from being brief and self-limiting to a severe pseudo-membranous colitis with possible gut perforation and death. Those who are most at risk of the severest disease are the elderly with serious co-existing disease.

Although 3% of adults carry it in their guts most cases of C. diff. diarrhoea arise from cross infection from others who have excreted spores in their faeces which have been ingested. The spores are resistant to alcohol.

The main action we can take to reduce this disease is to be judicious in the use of broad spectrum antibiotics. Antibiotics should be used only when absolutely necessary. In our hospital there is a policy governing their use for certain conditions and they are automatically stopped after five days. Certain broad spectrum antibiotics can only be prescribed with the permission of a Consultant microbiologist. Secondly

---

Wash Hands with soap and water

1. Before starting work
2. After using toilet
3. Before eating
4. When visibly contaminated
5. After finishing work

Use alcohol hand rub

1. On entering ward or clinical area
2. Between patients
3. Before and after aseptic procedures

Use the same hand movements as for washing
Only use if hands are visibly clean

Hand cleaning: use the same hand movements when washing or using alcohol solution   Should only take 15 to 30 seconds

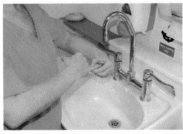

1. Take off rings and watches and ensure bare below elbows.

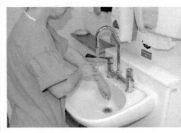

2. Turn on taps and wet hands thoroughly.

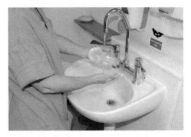

3. Generous soap application, enough to cover hands completely.

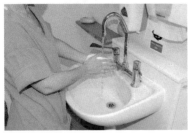

4. Rub palms together to generate a good lather.

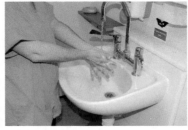

5. Rub palm onto back of hand with fingers interlocked.

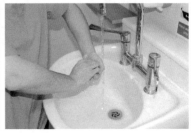

6. Cup hands together to clean back of fingers and nails.

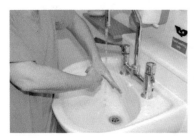

7. Scrub thumbs with a twisting motion, making sure you get into pits.

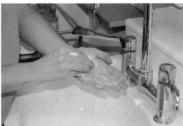

8. Rub the tip of fingers against palm of hands in a circular motion (to clean nails).

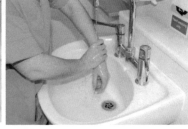

9. Wash the wrists.

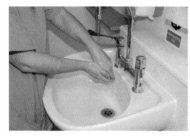

10. Rinse hands thoroughly.

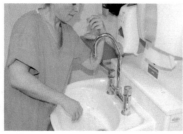

11. Turn off taps with elbows.

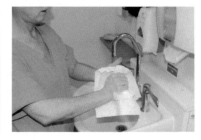

12. Dry hands with a single use towel.

14

patients who have C. diff. should be isolated and barrier nursed and thirdly we should be meticulous about hand hygiene on the wards and if there is a patient around who has diarrhoea then hands should be washed with soap and water rather than using alcoholic hand rub, as the spores are alcohol resistant.

When carrying out procedures on patients you should wear apron, mask, goggles and gloves, collectively known as Personal Protective Equipment (PPE). Such procedures include changing dressings or IV lines on the ward or cannulating patients There is no evidence to show that anything more is necessary when carrying out minor surgery, such as dental extraction or biopsy, in the outpatient facility. However the house rules or custom may be to wear a full theatre gown for these procedures, in which case you should abide by them.

Putting on Protective Equipment (PPE) (apron, mask, goggles and gloves)

PPE should be worn to reduce the chance of you spreading infection from one patient to another and for your own protection. It should be used when carrying out procedures on patients which involve contact with saliva, blood or when attending to any open wound. It should also be worn when entering a room where a patient is being nursed in isolation because they have an infection.

You should pay attention to putting on your PPE and taking it off in the correct order.

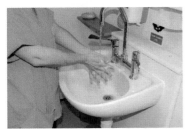

1. Clean hands with alcohol hand rub or soap and water.

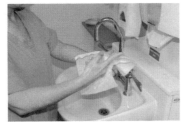

2. Dry hands; ensure they are completely dry.

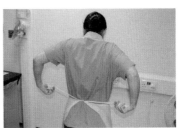

3. Put on apron- place over head and tie at back.

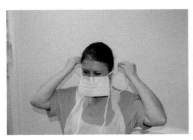

4. Put on mask ensuring a good seal between mask and face.

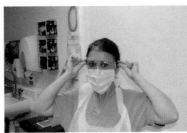

5. Put on goggles.

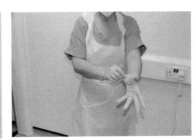

6. Put on gloves.

Removing PPE

Assume the PPE is contaminated and remove in the correct order.

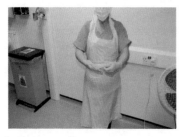

1. Remove gloves; grasp one glove and peel back carefully.

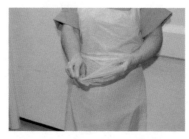

2. Place second glove in gloved hand and pull back glove with first glove inside it.

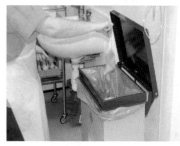

3. Discard in clinical waste bin.

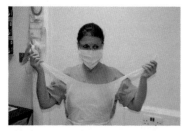

4. Remove apron by breaking ties at back of neck and waist.

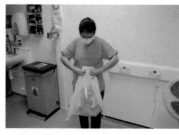

5. Pull apron away only touching its inside ; fold into a bundle.

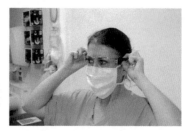

6. Remove goggles holding arms only.

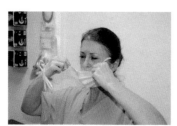

7. Remove mask by breaking straps at the side and pulling away from face. Do not touch the front of the mask.

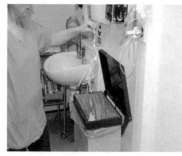

8. Discard into clinical waste bin.

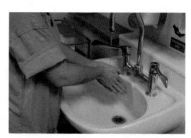

9. Clean hands when all PPE is removed.

8. Inoculation (needlestick) Injuries

All clinical workers in dental surgery are at risk of needlestick injury. The greatest risk is from the penetration of the operator's or assistant's skin with a hollow bore needle contaminated with blood (or saliva). Within the term 'needlestick injury' we include skin penetration by any sharp instrument, wire, broken glass, sharp tooth or even bone, contamination of the operator's skin at the site of a cut or abrasion or the contamination of mucous membrane of the mouth or eye.

The potential risk is from the blood borne viruses, and the stakes can be high. There is a risk of becoming HIV positive or a carrier of hepatitis B or C virus, with death from liver cirrhosis or cancer a possibility. In addition, a chronic carrier will have to give up all 'exposure prone procedures' which includes nearly all of clinical dentistry. Surgeons or nurses in training, including dental, are at the highest risk so it is wise to know as much about this hazard and how to reduce the risks before you start, especially as it has been estimated that about 80 % of injuries are preventable.

The risk is not limited to just these three well known conditions. There is also a risk from human T lymphotrophic retroviruses, hepatitis D and G virus, cytomegalovirus, Epstein Barr Virus, parvovirus, transfusion-transmitted virus, West Nile Virus, malarial parasites and prion agents which may cause spongiform encephalopathies.

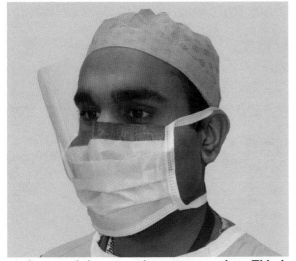

A face mask incorporating eye protection. This is cumbersome; you may prefer wide rimmed glasses.

How to avoid needlestick injuries

1. Wear gloves for all clinical procedures where hands might be contaminated with blood or saliva

2. Cover cuts or skin abrasions with a waterproof dressing before donning gloves

3. Never resheath needles. Remove needles from syringes and blades from knives with forceps and always away from you

4. When carrying out minor oral surgery with an assistant, but no scrub nurse, the surgeon should dispose of sharps into the sharps bin at the end to avoid risk to the nursing staff. The sharps bin should be disposed of when ¾ full

5. In theatre the scrub nurse places all sharps on a sharps pad which is sealed and placed in the sharps bin

6. Surgical knives should be passed between scrub nurse and surgeon in a bowl

7. During surgery retract with instruments not hands

8. Double glove for high risk procedures such as placing wire around teeth. This does not avoid the risk of skin puncture but may reduce the volume inoculated if this happens

9. Change gloves if punctured. Indicator gloves worn as an inside layer may show up a puncture

10. Wear large rim spectacles or a mask to prevent eye contamination when operating. There is a small risk of seroconverting from blood or saliva splashed into the eye. There is no risk from contamination of intact skin

---

So what is the degree of risk? There have been many studies which have attempted to assess the risk to health care workers from needlestick injuries. The Health Protection Agency has estimated that the risk of infection from a needlestick injury where the patient carries Hepatitis B virus (HBV) is about 1:3, for Hepatitis C (HCV) 1:30 and HIV 1:300. However, this degree of risk is very approximate as there are many variables; these include the depth of the wound caused,

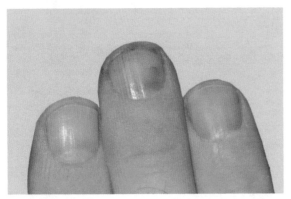

Blood on fingers after an orthognathic operation. Blood borne viruses will not penetrate intact skin but they will if the skin is damaged. There is a high risk of glove puncture when using wires or if the patient has fixed orthodontic appliances. Use double gloves.

Patient (donor) risk assessment after needlestick injury

Enquire about:-

Known or unknown blood borne virus (BBV) status

Risk factors for BBV

↑ risk of HIV sub-Saharan Africa

↑ risk of HIV homosexual, IV drug users, HIV mothers or sexual partners

↑ risk HCV received unscreened blood or plasma products (prior to 1991 & 1985 respectively in UK

the degree of infectivity of the donor blood or saliva i.e. 'e' or surface antigen for Hepatitis B or viral load for HIV.

Although Hepatitis B is the most infectious the good news is that if you have been immunised and you are one of the 90% who respond with a good antibody level then your risk should be zero. The 1:3 risk quoted above is for a non-immune recipient and an HBeAg+ve donor. If you have not responded to immunisation (usually obese men first immunised at over 40 years of age) then the risk of seroconverting can be reduced with post exposure prophylaxis with immunoglobulin.

Least infectious is HIV. The risk can be reduced by use of post exposure prophylaxis. There have been few proven cases of transmission to health care workers and these are mostly where the worker has received a deep wound with a hollow needle used for taking blood from an infected patient in the latter stage of the disease when they have a high viral load. As with all blood borne virus transmission the risk of mucous membrane contamination is much less than with a skin puncture wound.

Most dangerous is Hepatitis C. Although prevalence in the UK is only about 0.02 % of the population the seroconversion rate from accidental inoculation from a Hepatitis C carrier is greater than that of HIV.

What to do when you sustain a needlestick injury when operating

You should stop operating, un-scrub and remove gloves and wash the injured part thoroughly with soap or chlorhexidine and running water. Bleeding should be encouraged. If your eye, mouth or nose have been splashed with blood or blood contaminated saliva they should be washed with copious amounts of running water. The on duty manager or your superior should be informed.

Your employer will have a policy and procedure to follow which should be available in the operating theatre or outpatient clinic. This will probably be posted on the hospital intranet site available from all computers. The Occupational Health Department

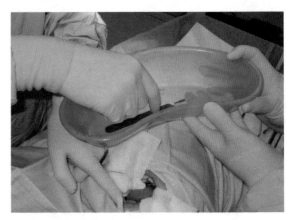

Scrub nurse passes knife to surgeon in a dish.

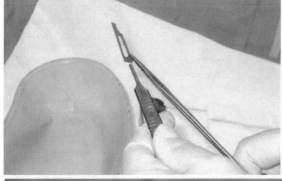

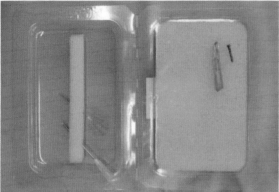

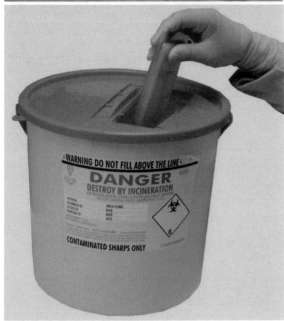

Blades are removed with a needle holder and placed on a sharps pad which is sealed before disposal. A disposable scalpel is even safer (below.)

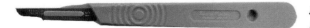

should be contacted for detailed advice. If it is closed you will probably find that the service is provided by the Accident and Emergency department.

The advice will be along the lines that the patient (if identified) should be told of the mishap and reassured that there is negligible risk to them. A risk assessment of the patient for the blood borne viruses should be made from previous history and habits. If the risk is considered significant then a blood sample should be taken for HIV, Hepatitis B and C. Of course the patient must give consent for this but in practice this is seldom refused. The patient's serum will be tested as soon as possible.

The requirement for specific prophylactic treatment will be determined by the initial risk assessment and the immune status of the staff member for Hepatitis B. If the initial assessment reveals negligible risk then no action is needed, but if there is a significant risk then the patient's serum should be tested as soon as possible and the injured staff member should start on antiviral treatment for HIV. They should commence a 28 day course of truvada (Tenofovir disoproxil and Emtricitabine), one tablet twice daily and kaletra (Lopinavir and Ritonavir), 2 tablets twice daily. Medication should be started within one hour of exposure but there may be a limited benefit if delayed for up to 72 hours. The medication will be available

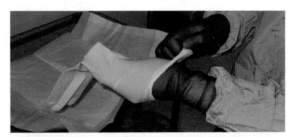

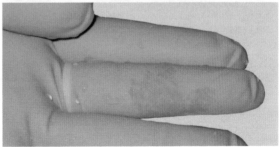

For high risk procedures such as when using wires 'indicator' gloves can be worn beneath normal gloves. If outer glove is penetrated moisture will show green.

19

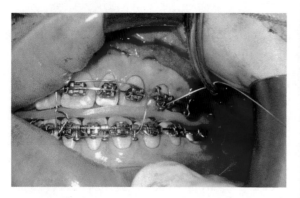

Wiring the jaws with fixed orthodontic appliances produces the greatest risk of glove penetration, as in this orthognathic case. Wear double gloves.

from the Occupational Health Department or from the Accident and Emergency Department.

These drugs can have significant systemic side effects but can be stopped if the patient is subsequently found to be HIV negative. It has been estimated that it may reduce the risk of acquiring HIV by as much as 80%. If the staff member is among those who do not have Hepatitis B immunity then they can be started on Hepatitis B immunoglobulin.

There is no effective post exposure prophylaxis for Hepatitis C. If, on testing, the patient is shown to be negative for Hepatitis C RNA then no action is taken. As soon as is practical after an inoculation injury blood should be taken from the victim. This is not tested but is stored for two years as evidence. However, if the patient turns out to have HIV then the staff member should be tested at three months and if they have Hepatitis C then they should be tested at 6 weeks, 3 and 6 months after the injury. If they have become infected they will have HCV antibodies for about six months but later detection of Hepatitis C RNA indicates an active or chronic infection and a state of infectivity to others.

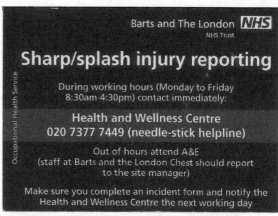

You may be given a sharps injury advice card to keep in your wallet.

9. Day Surgery

More patients will be admitted to the Day Surgery Unit than to the overnight stay surgical wards. Day surgery is popular with patients because they generally prefer not to have to stay in hospital if it can be avoided. However, the main reason for the expansion of day surgery is because it is cheaper.

Much day surgery within our speciality will be dento-alveolar in nature and, although the vast majority of it can be carried out under local anaesthetic in an outpatient department, sometimes with sedation, on those very few occasions where a general anaesthetic is desirable or demanded by the patient, it will usually be done in the day unit.

Most of these facilities will have a Consultant in overall charge of the facility, but for practical every-day running there will usually be a sister in charge. The unit will usually have facilities for patients to be seated prior to surgery and they will normally be recovered afterwards on a trolley on which they will be accommodated during the operation. The patients will normally walk in to the anaesthetic room. The whole flow of patients is organized to maximize efficiency and turnover.

Usually there will be an operating theatre suite within the facility itself. This decreases transportation time between cases but some may be situated adjacent to the main theatre complex, which allows the surgical team the greater flexibility of being able to mix day stay patients and inpatients on the same operating lists.

The most important consideration is choosing which patients and cases are suitable. The Royal College of Surgeons has published guidelines for this, and most hospitals will follow these or use criteria which are very similar. In some hospitals patients who require surgery will be sent to a Day Surgery Nurse, who will go through a pre-booking check list to confirm their suitability at the day of their initial outpatient consultation. Patients are given a pre-arranged date around which to organize their affairs. This should have no chance of being cancelled, as is sometimes the case of inpatient appointments due to emergency cases being admitted to the beds.

In most cases patients will be given a date for day surgery when they attend the outpatient clinic for their first consultation. They should undergo the pre-admission 'clerking' by a staff nurse so that when the

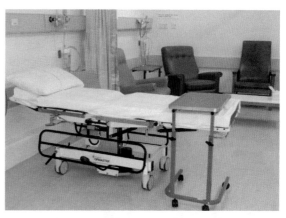

Most patients wait in chairs and transfer to a trolley before surgery; they stay on the same trolley for surgery and recovery

patient arrives on the day unit there is little for the trainee to do other than to greet the patient, ask if they have any more questions, confirm their consent for operation and familiarize themselves with each case before participating in the list as surgeon or assistant.

Day Surgical operations should take no longer than half an hour and be performed by a fully trained surgeon i.e. a Consultant or Staff Surgeon. A surgeon in training may perform day surgery in their final two years of training. This does not mean that someone more junior such as trainees cannot assist or operate under supervision but they must not be the most senior surgeon present in the theatre. All dento-alveolar surgery can potentially be carried out on a day case basis. Some may be more complex than others, but it has been shown that case complexity itself should be no bar to surgery under anaesthetic as day stay or, for that matter, for local anaesthesia.

Most limitations on a patient being suitable for day surgery will be related to their social circumstances and their medical status. The patient should reside within 45 minutes' travelling time of the hospital, have an adult to accompany them home, preferably (but not necessarily) driving them in a private car, and have a responsible adult to be with them throughout the night and the following 24 hours.

The American Society of Anaesthetists in 1962 devised the Physical Status Classification System range from a Grade 1 (fit and healthy) to Grade 6 (dead). For day surgery the patient must be ASA grade 1 or 2, although most of our day patients will be ASA grade 1.

Very occasionally patients booked for day surgery will need to stay overnight. This may occur because they have needed opiate analgesia and remain drowsy by the early evening or because they bled post-operatively. Occasionally a patient may arrive and, contrary to advice, has not arranged for a suitable adult to accompany them home, or may even intend to drive home themselves. These matters are always checked by the nurse when the patient arrives and if a bed is not available to accommodate them overnight or they announce that they are going anyway the anaesthetist will refuse to proceed. Of course it is a matter of liberty that the patient can do what they like afterwards but the advice having been given and the fact that it has been refused should be carefully documented in the patient's notes.

Patients who are grossly obese may have an airway problem after a general anaesthetic and so must be carefully monitored post-operatively. It is therefore considered unsafe to do day surgery under anaesthetic for patients whose body mass index is above 35. The index is a tool for indicating weight status in adults. It is worked out by the staff nurse at the pre clerking or booking clinic from the patient's weight and height using a chart.

The success of day surgery depends on good post-operative analgesia. In practical terms this involves infiltration of long acting local anaesthetic, Bupivacaine 0.5% with 1:200,000 Adrenaline adjacent to the operation site; this will give 6 to 8 hours of

Body Mass Index or BMI
For adults over 20 years old:
Below 18.5   = Underweight
18.5 – 24.9   = Normal
25.0 – 29.9   = Overweight
30.0 and over   = Obese
BMI =   weight in kilograms
(height in metres) X (height in metres) (but usually estimated from a chart)

$$BMI = \frac{\text{weight in kilograms}}{(\text{height in metres}) \times (\text{height in metres})}$$

analgesia. Diclofenac may be given before, during or after surgery; the slow release formulation should give 12 hours of comfort. This is usually followed up by Ibuprofen 400mgs t.d.s. orally with the advice to the patient that this is taken regularly for the first three days as pain is better anticipated with analgesia rather than reacted to.

Children need special consideration for day surgery. Most of the work will be dento-alveolar and much of it will be related to orthodontics, such as the removal of supernumerary teeth, uncovering of impacted canines for bracketing etc. Children should have separate ward and recovery facilities to adults with paediatric trained nurses to look after them. This may be provided in a special part of the day unit dedicated to children or, as in our own hospital, a day stay area of the paediatric unit. Children should preferably be near the beginning of the list to avoid an unnecessary prolonged period of pre-operative starving, and topical local anaesthetic such as lidocaine/prilocaine (EMLA®) or tetracaine (AMETOP®) should be placed over a prominent vein as soon as they arrive so that induction of anaesthesia can be painless and pleasant.

ASA grading
1. Normal healthy patient
2. Patient with mild systemic disease
3. Patient with severe systemic disease
4. Patient with severe systemic disease that is a constant threat to life
5. Moribund patient who is not expected to survive without the operation
6. Declared brain-dead patient whose organs are being removed for donor purposes

10. <u>The Ward: its Staff and Routines</u>

You will be involved in admitting a number of patients into the hospital ward. However, as a speciality only a small proportion of the patients we treat will need this. Indeed the majority of the patients receiving surgery will have it carried out on an outpatient basis.

Each ward has a sister or charge nurse in overall control with any number of registered nurses beneath, known as staff nurses. Each patient admitted should have a named nurse who will be in charge of their nursing care. On admission this nurse takes a full history; it is her job to know the patient in detail and to give a personalized nursing service. Obviously one nurse cannot be on duty for 24 hours so that when there is a change in shift there is 'a change over' and the nurse hands over the care of the patient to the new nurse, often by physically visiting the patients' beds.

In practice the patient turn over on acute surgical wards is very high and together with staffing problems

it is common for the named nurse to change frequently so it is not unusual to arrive on the ward and find that a particular patient's nurse is 'new to the ward' or 'just come on' and doesn't know much about the patient. Therefore the medical staff must maintain constant vigilance to ensure that the nurses looking after the patient know the important details about each particular client. The trained registered nurses will be supported on the ward by healthcare support workers who perform a non-specialized service such as helping with washing, bed making and distribution of meals.

At the end of each bed is written the name of the Consultant or speciality who is in overall charge of that patient. There should also be a folder containing the nursing notes, the drugs chart and the temperature and other 'observation' charts.

The history taken by the nurse is designed for her to become cognizant of all the patient's problems, treatment and concerns and expectations. She will also take particular note of the social background and details of home support after the patient has been discharged from the ward. There will be a nursing 'care plan' which will be written in the nursing notes. We frequently find that the nurses are so busy writing all this that there is inadequate time for attending to the patients. However when it comes to writing reports and statements sometime after the event it is often the nursing notes which are the most complete, legible and useful.

The nurses will also be responsible for recording certain observations for the patients, on observation charts in the folder. These 'vital signs' include blood pressure, temperature and pulse. There will also be other specific observations, which may be requested in certain circumstances. In particular a fluid balance chart will record the oral and parenteral intake of fluid and urine output; neurological observations will be made for patients who have received head injuries, or eye observations for patients who have received surgery for peri-orbital fractures.

Nursing shifts usually change at 7.30am, 2pm and 9pm and you should ensure that you visit the ward at least once during every nursing shift. In practical terms this must include a formal ward round of the patients in the morning with the Consultants or the Specialist Registrar, a visit to the patients at the end of the working day (after 5.00 p.m.) and another short visit

<u>*Indications for Ward admission in OMFS*</u>

1. Major surgery requiring specialized post op surgical care

2. Multiple injuries

3. Mandibular fractures awaiting urgent theatre

4. Mid face fractures for post-operative care or observation

5. Head injuries for observation where there has been loss of consciousness or nausea

6. Routine Surgery under GA with a co existing medical problem such as poorly controlled diabetes, cardiac disease or bleeding diathesis

7 Routine surgery which cannot be done as day stay because patient:-

 a. lives a long distance away

 b. will not be accompanied home

 c. will be alone for the first 24 hours post surgery

 d. has body mass index + 35

after the night shift have come on at about 10 pm. In the case of the occasional patient who is in hospital for a prolonged stay and in whom there is little change in their condition, the last two visits will be very short. For post-operative cases, particularly major ones, it will be more prolonged and the senior staff will probably visit the patient twice or more per day with you. In either case you should ensure that you are there to receive and understand their instructions for management.

It is important that sufficient information is passed onto colleagues for the patients to be looked after adequately when you are off duty. 'Handover' is best carried out at the patient's bedside but this may not always be practical. Information given verbally can be supplemented by a written note. It is particularly useful to pass on a written management plan at weekends.

Prior to operation the patient's named nurse will be responsible for pre-operative preparation. She will ensure the consent form has been completed, that the anesthetist has seen the patient and, if you are unaware of any specific anxieties that the patient may have, they will make sure that they are dissipated or communicated to the surgical team as appropriate. The nurse will accompany the patient to the operating theatre and will collect them from the theatre recovery room after the operation.

When the patient is fit to be discharged from the hospital, the named nurse will arrange for the outpatient appointment to be made and will communicate with the District Nurse should any nursing be required at home, for example change of dressings. They will also communicate with relatives to arrange collection of the patient from the ward.

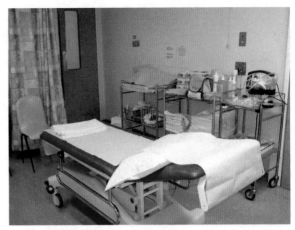

The ward will have a treatment room where patients can be examined in privacy and minor procedures carried out.

In addition to the trained nurses and healthcare support workers there are many other professionals, based on, or visiting the wards, who participate in the patient's care. The ward clerk will make sure that the records are present for the admission if the hospital does not yet use electronic records. She will collate the results of investigations such as blood tests. When they have been signed by the professional staff, to confirm that they have been seen, she will file them in the notes. Once a day the ward pharmacist will visit; she will check the drug chart and make sure that the prescribed drugs are available. In addition she is a valuable additional safe guard against prescribing errors; if there are any doubts or queries she will write them on the charts. Doubts by the pharmacist or nurse about drugs or their dosage should always be considered very seriously.

Each morning a phlebotomist will visit the ward to take blood for routine tests etc. In order for them to help you it will therefore be necessary to make sure requests have been made through the clinical records system the night before. A physiotherapist will visit each ward; they usually visit patients on the request of the named nurse. It is unlikely in OMFS that patients will have locomotor problems and need help with mobilization, but post-operative patients, particularly those who have had pre-existing chest disease or are smokers, will be given chest physiotherapy on request.

The dietician will visit the ward to give advice and prescribe nutritional supplements to patients who are having difficulties with eating. In our speciality there may be the occasional patient who has inter-maxillary fixation or more likely patients having enteral tube

---

Written management plan for week end handover

1. Diagnosis

2. Any important medical history

3. 1-3 line summary of progress since admission

4. Investigations needed & if requested

5. Procedures to be done, when & by whom

5. Discharge summary should be written in advance

(Gibbons & Khattak. British Dental Journal 2005)

Checks before a patient can be discharged

1. Patient can eat & drink

2. Has passed urine

3. Apyrexial

4. Adequate pain control with oral analgesics

5. Is self caring or has adequate help

6. Has transport home or can be accompanied

feeding if they are 'nil by mouth' following oral reconstruction consequent on ablative cancer surgery.

Most of those admitted for Oral or Maxillofacial Surgery will be patients receiving ablative cancer operations, who need specialized post-operative care, trauma patients, those receiving Orthognathic Surgery or those who have severe oro-facial sepsis. Some patients may be admitted because they have co-existing medical problems and are having a general anaesthetic, for example poorly controlled diabetics, or patients with cardiac disease or bleeding diathesis. Sometimes there may be social reasons, such as having no one to take them home after surgery or they live a long way from the hospital. Some patients may be admitted because they are too obese for a general anaesthetic as a day stay (body mass index +35).

Most patients will be fit to go home when they are able to eat, drink, pass urine, their pain has been controlled and they are able to get home and look after themselves or have someone else to help. If they do not and they are infirm the social workers may need to be involved and an occupational therapy assessment may be needed to ascertain what level of support they need. This should ideally be predicted in advance in order to avoid unnecessary delay and the bed being 'blocked' by a patient who does not need acute surgical care anymore.

You should ensure that the patient has an outpatient review appointment (but only if necessary), that appropriate medication has been prescribed (particularly analgesics if they have had surgery), and post-operative instructions given. The patient's GP should be informed of the discharge by completing the electronic discharge document on a hospital computer.

11. <u>Preparation for Theatre</u>

Preparation for a routine cold operation will start in the outpatient clinic with the discussion between surgeon and patient about the indications, contraindications and alternatives to surgery. A consent form will need to be completed and signed as an adjunct to this process. If the surgery is to be carried out under local anaesthetic it will usually be carried out in the outpatient department, and if under general anaesthetic as a day stay, but a minority of patients will be admitted to the ward.

At this stage the patient will usually be given a date for surgery out of the diary and be seen by a registered nurse who will carry out the process often called 'pre-clerking' or 'care planning', which is designed to ensure that the patient is fully prepared, that the appropriate investigations are carried out and that they know what to expect and where to come and when. If day surgery is planned the nurse will check that their physical health and social circumstances concord with the accepted criteria for day surgery.

This will involve going through, with the patients, a fairly complicated care plan document, which includes a detailed assessment of their current and previous medical and social history, a systems review of symptoms they may have which might indicate any underlying cardiac or respiratory disease, and a social history which might have a bearing on their discharge from hospital and post-operative care after they no longer need nursing care on the ward. The assessment will usually include routine observations such as blood pressure, pulse, height, weight and body mass index. Current medication will be listed. The patient will be given instructions about not eating for six hours prior to surgery and not drinking for four.

Investigations will be ordered by the nurse under a protocol which will almost certainly follow the guidelines of the National Institute for Health & Care Excellence (NICE). This should ensure that no one should present on the day of surgery without the essential investigations having been done and checked, and resources should not have been wasted on requesting unnecessary tests.

It is usual practice that patients are admitted to hospital on the day of their surgery rather than the day before. On the morning of surgery there will be further checks to be made by the admitting nurse. It will need

Investigation	_Indication_
ECG	Pre existing cardiac or respiratory disease Smoker over 40 Anyone over 60
Chest X Ray	Is almost never needed but may be requested if there is existing cardiac or respiratory disease
Full blood count	Over 60 Anyone for major surgery with significant blood loss More minor surgery with some blood loss with history of cardiac disease
Urea & electrolytes	Renal disease Diabetics Taking diuretics
Serum glucose	Diabetics On steroids Severe sepsis
Coagulation screen	Anti coagulants (INR) Liver disease Family or past history of problem bleeding
Sickle/ Hb. electrophoresis	Ethnic groups at risk if not previously tested or no history of previous anaesthetic if counselled and consented. North African, West African, South/sub Saharan African, Afro Caribbean, Eastern Mediterranean, Middle Eastern, Asian.

Pre-operative investigations in OMFS

United Lincolnshire Hospitals **NHS**

NHS Trust

Integrated Care Pathway for Day Care or Short Stay Patients

Patient NHS No

Patient Name

This pathway is for patients aged 16 years and over identified as requiring a day surgical procedure with a length of stay of less than 23 hours

Specialty		TCI
Consultant		
Proposed Procedure		
Actual Procedure		

General Anaesthesia	Regional Anaesthesia	LA/ IV +/- Sedation

Signature Record

All members of staff who are using this Integrated Care Pathway should use black ink and complete this section. You can then use initials when recording care.

Print Name	Job Title	Bleep No or Ext	Signature	Initials

Allergies / Sensitivities	Yes	No
Specify and list reaction		

Does the patient have an allergy / sensitivity associated with latex? If yes, inform the following
□ Theatres □ Surgeon □ Ward □ Anaesthetist

This Integrated Care Pathway is intended as a guide to care only and does not replace clinical judgement.
Copyright © 2007 United Lincolnshire Hospitals NHS Trust

Created by ULHT Day Care and Surgical Team
Day Care or Short Stay ICP V11 Jun 07 / Document number: ULHT-G/2007/022 Review date: Apr 09   Page 1 of 12

The 12 page care plan booklet which is completed by a nurse in the presence of the patient as part of the pre admission for surgery process. Bureaucracy rules!

to be confirmed when they last ate or drank; they will need to be fitted with an identity band, and the consent form will be returned and signed. The patient will be dressed in a theatre gown, decorative finger rings will be taped, and dentures or spectacles removed and kept in a safe place, usually the bed side locker. Patients will be seen by the anaesthetist for a pre-operative assessment and by someone from the surgical team who will need to find out if there are any further questions or explanations which should be attended to and this will be confirmed on the consent form. If the operation is outside the mouth the operation site should be marked with a skin marking pen and the admission document signed to confirm that this has been done. You should ensure that you visit the ward or day unit with the surgeon in charge and familiarise yourself with their case history and examine them if you have not already had the opportunity to do so.

Pre-operative investigations are not all done as a routine; there is no point in carrying out a special test at some inconvenience and expense if it has a small chance of providing an abnormal result which may not change the management of the patient. There is also the potential problem that false positive results may postpone surgery and lead to more unnecessary tests and lead to inappropriate treatment.

Once the theatre is ready, with both surgeon and anaesthetist present, the senior nurse in change of the list will inform the theatre receptionist who will send a porter to the ward to fetch the patient. The patient will return with their named nurse and will be booked into the theatre by the receptionist. A nurse from the appropriate theatre will then come and receive the patient from the named nurse. She will ask the patient to confirm verbally their name and what procedure they are having carried out. She will also check the patient's name and hospital number on a band, which has been placed round their wrist as soon as they enter the ward. This is to ensure that the patient ends up in the correct theatre for the correct operation.

Once in the anaesthetic room the surgeon may wish to confirm the patient's identity and pass the time of day with them. The anaesthetist will again check the patient's wrist band and then start the anaesthetic assisted by the operating department practitioner. Once the anaesthetic has been administered the patient will be transferred to the operating theatre and the operation commences. You should scrub and participate in the surgery in whatever manner you are instructed to by the senior surgeon present.

12. <u>Consent for Hospital Treatment</u>

It needs to be emphasized, as it is often not well understood, that consent for treatment in hospital is much more than the placement of the signature on a form. Consent is the process whereby the patient is informed about what treatment can be provided, what the alternatives are and what are the risks and their side-effects of each treatment as well as the benefits. There should include a discussion about the consequences of no treatment. The patient must understand what is being offered and be capable of absorbing the information and making choices offered to them. The consent form is a useful adjunct to this process but is not the be all and end all that many in the hospital consider it to be. Good clinical notes are as important.

The standards which are used in an acute NHS trust for obtaining consent are important to the National Health Service Litigation Authority (NHSLA) which provides indemnity to NHS trusts under their Clinical Negligence Scheme for Trusts (CNST) scheme. The hospital trust will pay a premium to the NHSLA which

<u>*Sources of Guidance on Consent*</u>

These four organisations have all published informative guidance on consent issues and the law. You will almost certainly have read one or more of them. If not you should do so now. They can be downloaded from their web sites as PDF files.

General Medical Council: Consent: patients and doctors making decisions together

Medical Protection Society: An MPS Essential Guide to Consent

General Dental Council: Principles of Patient Consent

Dental Protection: Consent to Dental Treatment, The principles and their application

In addition we commend the following papers:

Informed consent: the dawning of a new era. N. Khalique. Editorial British Journal of Oral and Maxillofacial Surgery. 53 (2015) 479-484.

Consent - a new era begins. L D'Cruz & H Kaney. British Dental Journal 2015: 219: 57-59

<u>*Some Principles of Consent*</u>

The decision must be the patient's.

Patient must have the capacity to make a decision; it must be assumed that a patient does have the capacity unless it is established that he does not.

The patient should be warned of any material risks of proposed treatment and of alternatives.

The doctor should be aware which particular risks the patient would regard as material.

Children under 16 may have the capacity to consent to treatment.

A parent can consent to treatment for a child.

A person aged 16 can be presumed to have capacity to consent.

No one can give consent on behalf of another adult.

Patient should be told of the diagnosis, proposed treatment, its risks & complications, alternative treatments, their risks and complications and the consequence of no treatment.

Patient must give consent voluntarily.

may be discounted by up to 30% if best practice is carried out when they assess the Trust every 2 to 3 years. Consenting patients for treatment is only one of the many parameters which will be investigated but it is among the most important. The gold standard is that the patient's consent is obtained by the clinician who is able to perform the procedure; this is what happens in practice in most cases in the best OMFS departments. However, failing this, consent should be obtained from somebody who has been trained to do it and is able to discuss the benefits, risks and side-effects of the procedure and its alternatives.

The consent process should involve making sure that the patient is aware of any material risks involved in the recommended treatment and of any variant or alternative treatments. The surgeon should be aware if that particular patient will be likely to attached significance to any particular risk. We believe, therefore, that obtaining consent for surgery is not a *[handwritten notes]* Warned about post op swelling + paraesthesia absolute centres. Possible numbness of lower lip due to potential nerve damage. Which may need to postpone surgery if swelling is down at the time + not visible.

Warnings of complications should be recorded in the patient's notes.

Thank you for asking me to see Mr   concerning the swelling in his lower lip.

Clinically this looks like a mucous extravasation cyst due to trauma from his teeth. I have advised him that this will continue to recur if it is not removed so we are making arrangements to carry this out under local anaesthetic. I have advised Mr   that his lip will be swollen, sore and uncomfortable for about a week afterwards and there is a small risk of some numbness of the vermilion of the lower lip due to the proximity of the small nerves which supply sensation to it.

Yours sincerely

It is helpful to mention them in the letter to the GP and send a copy to the patient.

suitable job to be delegated to a new trainee.

Consent is usually, and properly, obtained from the patient at the initial outpatient appointment; the discussion over the treatment is part of the consent process. This should be done by the Consultant or Staff Surgeon who is seeing the patient in the clinic. Comprehensive notes, written at the time, provide evidence that a robust consenting process has been used. This is probably of as much use as the consent form itself. Properly written notes are augmented by letters back to the referring practitioner and it has been our practice to send copies of these letters to patients for their information.

It is also good practice to fill in the consent form itself at the initial outpatient visit when the decision to operate is made; this is sometimes varied for minor surgery carried out with local anaesthetic in the outpatient department. We believe it is unfair to ask a patient to sign a consent form just before major surgery where they may be anxious or frightened, especially when the discussion on which it is based was carried out a few weeks before. However, it is normal practice to reconfirm consent just before treatment by visiting the patient in the surgical admissions lounge or day unit and asking them if they have any further questions about their treatment. This is recorded on the consent form.

The forms used are fairly standard in acute NHS trusts; they are very far from perfect. It is also unfair to ask a patient to sign straight away in the clinic as

The Consent Forms

Form 1: Patient agreement to investigation or treatment

Form 2: For parental agreement investigation or treatment for a child or young person

Form 3: Patient/ parental agreement for investigation or treatment which does not require a general anaesthetic. (procedures where consciousness is not impaired)

Form 4: Form for adults who are unable to consent to investigation or treatment

there is too much on the form for them to read and it gives them insufficient time to digest the discussion that has taken place. Most patients, in our experience, do not bother to read the forms (often they don't have their spectacles with them). We prefer to fill in our part of a form and ask the patient to take it away to sign later and bring it back with them. However, about a third of patients forget to bring it back with them and we have often to fill out another.

In practice there are few problems with the consenting process. Initially you will be too inexperienced to consent patients for operation other than for very minor procedures such as a biopsy. Remember, the consent form itself should be written in terms that can be understood, so abbreviations and dental chartings should not be used. The forms themselves have a top copy of the information recorded by the clinician which tears off for the patient to keep a record of their own.

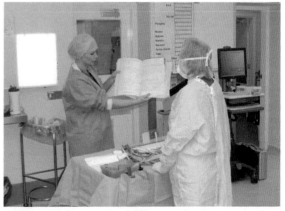

Nurses in theatre check the consent form to ensure the patient is getting the right operation.

The consent form 4 is used for adult patients who are unable to consent for treatment. This is slightly more complicated and those who treat such patients should be aware of the law and in particular the Mental Incapacity Act. Usually the Consultant will be dealing with all such cases in OMFS and these are very few in number. In our practice they are most frequently severe trauma cases where the patient is sedated and intubated when we arrive. Usually our job is first aid in the shape of a tracheostomy, arrest of haemorrhage, suturing of lacerations, the removal of loose teeth and stabilisation of facial fractures. In these circumstances only the urgent treatment should be carried out and it must be in the patient's best interest. In some hospitals the OMF surgeons provide a tracheostomy service for patients who are already intubated and ventilated and therefore unable to give consent; consent form 4 will be used in all these cases.

Right: Specimen Consent Form 1- Fractured Mandible, general anaesthetic

Below: Consent issues for some common operations

Procedure	Intended benefit	Serious or frequently occurring risk	Our comment
Surgical removal of impacted third molar tooth	To prevent further pain or infection	Numbness or tingling of lip or tongue, <u>probably</u> temporary	Risk of permanent numbness about 2% tongue 0.25% lip
Incisional biopsy of swelling in mouth	For diagnosis of swelling		No need to mention swelling, discomfort or bleeding on the form. The patient should be verbally warned of these but they are not risks; rather they are side effects to be expected and are not serious
Excisional biopsy of swelling	To remove the lump and for diagnosis		
Suture of laceration of face	To close wound to achieve best appearance	None (leave blank)	
Open reduction & fixation of fracture of zygoma (malar)	Restore contour of face, improve jaw movement, improve chance of recovery of face numbness, improve double vision	Bleed into eye socket	Very rare but should be mentioned as this can threaten vision

13. <u>Working in the Operating Theatre</u>

You will probably be involved in one or two operating 'lists' in theatre each week. You should expect to be able to 'scrub up' for most of the cases and at least assist. Hopefully you will be allowed to carry some simple dento-alveolar surgery under supervision, although the days when significant numbers of wisdom teeth were removed under general anaesthetic have now gone.

The operating theatre is the most expensive facility in the hospital. It is therefore important that things run smoothly and efficiently and you may be able to contribute to this. However, the main consideration in the theatre is patient safety and this does not equate easily with speed, so things often run frustratingly slowly.

You will find that the operating theatre suite will have many individual theatres. Usually, these will be dedicated to specific disciplines or groups. Orthopaedics usually has its own dedicated theatres with laminar air ventilation in which bacteria free filtered air is circulated under pressure into the operating site so that contaminated air is removed away from the patient. This may reduce the incidence of airborne infection which can be disastrous in joint replacement surgery.

Each theatre will have its own anaesthetic room where the patient is prepared and anaesthetised; a preparation ('prep') room where the instruments and other equipment are prepared and laid out on trolleys; a 'scrub' room where surgeons, assistants and nurses

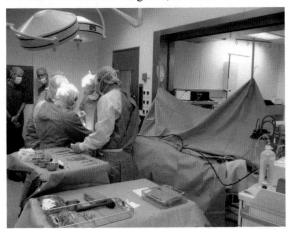

Theatre. The surgeon, assistant and scrub nurse wear sterile gowns; there is an unsterile 'runner' who fetches additional equipment.

wash their hands and put on gowns and gloves; there will be a 'dirty' area where instruments and drapes are taken after the operation and where pathology specimens from cancer surgery are taken to be orientated and pinned to a cork board for the pathologist. Somewhere in the suite there will also be store rooms, staff rest rooms, a kitchen, offices, a reception area and recovery rooms where the patients are taken immediately after surgery. All the theatres will be air conditioned with about 20 changes of air per hour so that airborne bacteria shed from the patients' or staff's skin or even from a dirty wound will be swiftly carried out.

A few days before each operating session a list of patients will have been prepared, usually by the Consultant's secretary or booked admissions team. The patients will be listed in order of booking time with their ages, hospital number and procedure recorded; there may be additional special theatre requirements added. The patients will have previously been screened by a nurse using a pre-assessment questionnaire to highlight medical or social problems which might impinge on their surgery or recovery from it. The surgery should have been explained and discussed with the surgeon, and a consent form signed. On the day of the surgery there will be further checks with the patient, in particular whether they have any last minute questions, whether they have starved for six hours (if they are to receive a general anaesthetic) and if someone is available to take them home (if a day case).

Each theatre in the suite will have a nurse in charge who may be a staff nurse or sister. When the anaesthetist and nurses are ready and the surgeon is known to have arrived, the nurse in charge will inform the theatre receptionist to send for the patient who will be escorted from the ward by a porter and a ward nurse. On arrival, the patient will be booked in at the theatre reception, their identity will be checked, both verbally and by looking at their wrist band, and the consent form will be checked. They will then be taken to the anaesthetic room.

The anaesthetic room contains all the equipment necessary to put the patient to sleep. The anaesthetist will be assisted by an Operating Department Practitioner (ODP). While the patient is being anaesthetised the surgical instruments are prepared in the 'prep' room by a nurse who has 'scrubbed'. This 'scrub nurse' will prepare the sterile instruments while

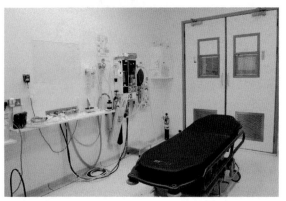
Anaesthetic room

an unsterile nurse, the 'runner', will hand things to her, touching only the unsterile part of the wrappings. The instruments used in any operation by a particular surgeon will be kept on a list in a card index in the theatre or computer so the nurse will know which instruments to prepare.

While the patient is in theatre all the staff involved in the operation will go through a World Health Organization (WHO) checklist which has three stages. The first, known as 'sign in', occurs before the anaesthetic is induced. Once 'sign in' has occurred the anaesthetic can commence. The ODP will draw up the drugs, unwrap and pass equipment and set up the monitoring equipment. When anaesthetised the patient can be transferred to the operating theatre and the operation commences. In the theatre itself the second stage of the WHO checklist, known as 'time out', takes place.

The surgeon and assistant should scrub while the patient is in the anaesthetic room so that they are ready to start as soon as the patient is on the table. During the operation the ODP will assist the anaesthetist while the scrub nurse passes instruments to the surgeon. The runner should remain in theatre and fetch equipment and instruments as required. The trainee should scrub and participate in the surgery in whatever manner instructed by the surgeon.

After the operation the final stage of the WHO checklist, known as 'sign out', is made. The senior surgeon will probably wish to write up the operating notes himself. For day cases a TTA (to take away) prescription should be made, usually on the computer, with an electronic discharge for the GP, usually completed by the trainee.

WHO Surgical Safety Checklist - Part 1 Sign in

Patient has confirmed:-

Identity, site, procedure, consent

Site marked/not applicable

Anaesthesia safety check completed

Pulse oximeter on patient and functioning

Does patient have:-

Known allergy: yes or no
Difficult airway/aspiration risk
No
Yes and equipment/assistance available
Risk of >500ml blood loss

No
Yes and adequate IV access and fluids
planned

There are several operating theatre rituals and conventions you will need to know about and adhere to; these are principally designed to reduce cross infection. The evidence for their efficacy is variable so you will find that there will be some slight variation between hospitals. You may find that some hospitals still require patients to remove all items of their own clothing, cover their hair and take off any jewellery. There is very little evidence to support these measures as an aid to cross infection so you will find most hospitals have abandoned these procedures. It is usual practice to tape rings to prevent their being dislodged and lost.

You will enter the theatre suite through a door directly into a changing room where you should change into an operating cotton suit; this will be freshly laundered but socially clean rather than sterile. You will find the appropriate sized suit on a shelf but some hospitals dispense them from a machine for which you will need your identity card. Outdoor shoes should be replaced with theatre footwear with impervious soles and these should be regularly cleaned. There is little evidence to show that leaving theatres in a surgical suit and returning without changing it increases infection rates, but it is usual to wear a coat or cover gown over the suit while outside the theatre. It is forbidden to wear a theatre suit outside the hospital building to avoid external contamination.

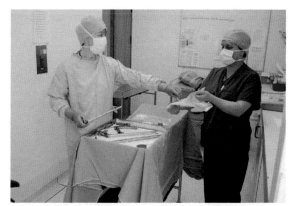

The sterile scrub nurse is preparing the instruments in the 'prep' room. The unsterile 'runner' is passing equipment by holding the unsterile outer wrapping.

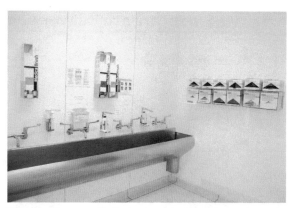

The scrub room. It is equipped with elbow operated taps. There are dispensers on the wall containing disposable nail brushes and sponges impregnated with chlorhexidine, PCMX or iodine and separate dispensers. Sterile gloves are on the wall.

The process of pre-operative hand washing and donning surgical gloves and sterile gown is known as 'scrubbing up'. Finger nails should be kept short, and the first wash of the day should include a thorough clean of the finger nails using a stick or brush. Thereafter the hands should be washed using chlorhexidine gluconate 4%, 7.5% Povidone iodine scrub solution or PCMX (Parachlorometaxylenol), using the technique previously described for 2 minutes. The supplied nail brushes should not be used on the skin as they can cause abrasions. Theatre gowns and drapes are now mostly disposable, as these are less permeable to epithelial cells and bacteria shed from staff or patients than the formerly used linen. Once you have scrubbed you should not touch any non-sterile surface or object. If you accidentally do touch something with your hand it is easier to put on a second glove than to change.

WHO Surgical Safety Checklist - Part 2 Time out

All team members introduce themselves by name and role

Surgeon, anaesthetist & nurse verbally confirm:-

Patient, Site, Procedure

Anticipated critical events:-

Surgeon reviews: Critical or unexpected steps, operative duration, anticipated blood loss

Anaesthesia review: any specific patient concerns
Nursing reviews: sterility confirmed, any equipment issues or other concerns

Has antibiotic prophylaxis been given in last 60 minutes? Yes/not applicable

Is essential imaging displayed? Yes/not applicable

You should find that it is normal practice in most theatres for all staff to wear protective caps. Again there is little evidence to support the need for this but adherence to this ritual is universal.

Staff who wear jewellery should remove it in theatre but a single wedding ring is usually not removed. It is thought that a ring worn beneath a glove does not contribute to cross infection although it may lead to an increase in glove perforation. False finger nails, however, do harbour pathogenic bacteria and should not be worn.

WHO Surgical Safety Checklist - Part 3 Sign out

Name of procedure recorded

Instrument, sponge & needle counts correct or not applicable

How the specimen is labeled

Whether there are any equipment problems to be addressed

Surgeon, anaesthetist & nurse review key concerns for recovery & management

---

14. <u>Scrubbing and Gowning</u>

Below is demonstrated the sequence of preparing yourself for surgery. This is called scrubbing up. It involves placing a sterile gown and gloves, opened, on the trolley, washing hands, putting on the gown followed by the gloves and getting someone to tie up the gown behind. Once scrubbed you must not touch anything unsterile with your hands or body.

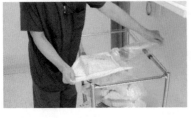

1. Tear open a gown pack touching only the outer wrap.

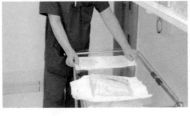

2. Open the glove packet touching only the outer wrap.

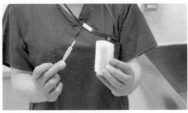

3. Antiseptic scrub solutions are impregnated into a sponge with a scrubbing brush & a nail cleaning tool.

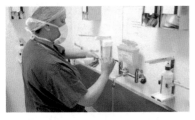

4. Clean beneath nails and scrub them but only for the first wash of the day. Do not brush other skin.

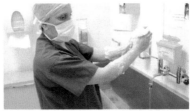

5. Use the same hand movements as on 'hand cleaning' section but go up towards elbows.

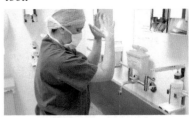

6. Turn off tap with elbows and let water drain off arms.

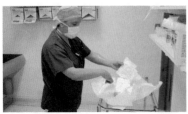

7. Open the gown pack; touch the outside of the inner wrap only. Take a paper towel.

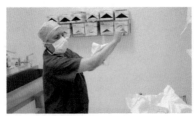

8. Dry the hands first moving up to elbows.

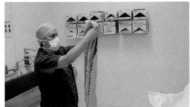

9. Take the gown, hold at the top and allow it to unroll; touch only the inside.

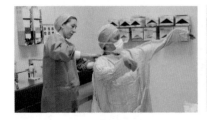

10. Push arms into gown. Runner pulls gown up arms from inside and ties gown behind.

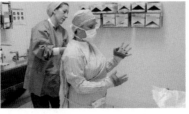

11. Hands protrude out of gown. We are going to use an 'open' technique to don gloves.

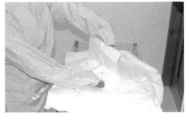

12. The glove packet being opened. They are packed with the cuff folded back.

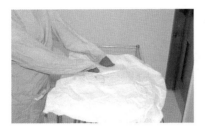

13. The cuff of the left glove is picked up, touching through the gown.

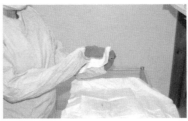

14. Fold the left glove over the left hand , pulling with the right hand touching the inside of the cuff area.

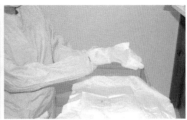

15. Pull the glove on.

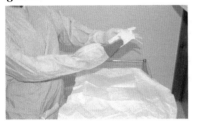

16. Pick up the second glove.

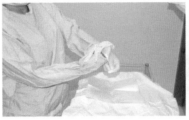

17. Pull on the right glove; you can touch this anywhere with the gloved left hand.

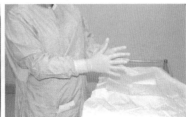

18. Complete.

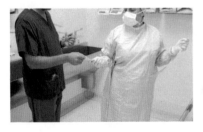

19. Now tie the waistband. Hand the card attached to the waistband to someone who is not scrubbed.

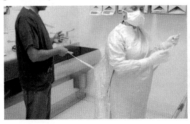

20. Twirl around so that the band goes around your waist and the back of the gown is closed.

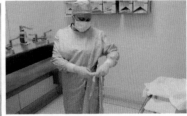

21. Take the other end of the band and tie it.

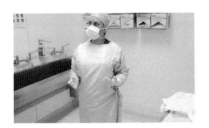

22. Ready for theatre.

15. <u>Routine Post-Operative Care</u>

Immediately following surgery the patient will be transferred from the operating theatre to the recovery room, within the operating theatre suite, when they are sufficiently awake. There they will be under the care of a single recovery nurse who will monitor the patient's welfare during recovery. The anaesthetist is responsible for handing over to the recovery staff and retains overall responsibility for the patient until they are transferred to the ward. When the recovery nurse is satisfied that the patient is sufficiently recovered to go back to the ward she will ask the anaesthetist for permission to do so and then call for a ward nurse and porter to take the patient. The recovery nurse will hand over to the ward nurse.

The surgical team, which includes you, should hand over any specific instructions or warnings concerning the surgery that the recovery nurse should know about.

After the operating session has finished you should visit the patient on the ward to check for any problems and make contact with the patient's named nurse to ensure they know of any special issues regarding their care. In most routine cases this contact will only need to be brief but very frequently patients may be admitted to non-specialist wards where the nurses are not experienced in looking after OMFS patients and you will need to explain the surgery to them. The anaesthetist will also visit the patient on the ward. This is usually a brief attendance to ensure that there is no problem with the airway and that the analgesia they have prescribed is sufficient.

Post-operative pain management is very important. Pain is much better anticipated than reacted to. It is important for you to check that this has been given and that the patients are comfortable.

It is desirable that the patient is visited at the end of the working day to check on them again and in the late evening after the night nursing staff have come on to ensure that they are familiar with the case. The surgeon should discuss what was done with the patient, any complications that might have arisen and the plan for recovery including anticipated time or date of discharge home.

The nurses should undertake routine observations of their breathing and respiratory rate, their consciousness, ability to speak and particularly any swelling or bleeding which might obstruct the airway. Temperature, pulse and blood pressure are routinely monitored and a note made of signs concerning their circulation such as colour. It is very desirable that the patient is encouraged to sit up, sit out of bed and walk, with aid if necessary, as early ambulation is desirable to prevent atelectasis (peripheral lung collapse) and venous thrombosis (see next chapter).

Each morning the surgical team should visit each patient on a ward round. You will go round with the Consultant or Specialist Registrar; this visit should include the patient's named nurse who will report on their progress. Pain, fluid intake (and output if it is a major case), eating, pain control should all be checked. The vital signs (pulse, blood pressure, temperature) should be checked from the patient's chart. Meticulous recording of these, by the nurses, is essential to facilitate awareness of early adverse changes. IV lines should be checked to ensure they are patent and if there is any sign of inflammation. If the patient is taking an adequate oral intake they may be removed. If surgical drains have been placed they should be checked to ensure they are working i.e. that they are not blocked or have lost their vacuum. If they are working but there has been little drainage they may be removed.

If the patient has pain adequately controlled, has passed urine, is eating and drinking, has a responsible adult to accompany them, then they can probably be discharged home. Follow up care should be discussed and arranged; possible complications and side effects should be discussed. Any medication to take home should be prescribed and a discharge pro-forma completed for the patient's General Medical Practitioner. You will have to do this, most probably on-line, usually with the patient being given a paper copy. This should include details of the problem, diagnosis, findings, follow up and medication.

Throughout the process you should record progress in the patient's notes including when they have been visited, by whom, changes in condition or management and the surgical plan.

16. <u>Post-Operative Complications</u>

A complication is an adverse event which may increase the morbidity of a patient following any treatment, most commonly, but not necessarily, a surgical operation. As surgeons we seek to minimise the risk of complications by good pre-operative planning, sound surgery and meticulous post-operative care. You will be part of this.

Complications may be classified as local or systemic and as immediate, delayed or late. We will discuss delayed or late systemic complications. Immediate complications will occur in the operating theatre where there will be a Consultant or Registrar present to deal with these and local complications, (i.e. at the operation site) will be part of your learning within the job. The next paragraph is the most important in this chapter.

We will thus be discussing mostly medical complications of surgery that OMFS patients are likely to sustain. The reason for discussing these is to allow you to understand what may go wrong and the principle of dealing with them. You will be part of the surgical team and will assist in post-operative management but at no stage must you, as a dentist, initiate the treatment of medical complications or manage them without the full intervention of the responsible Consultant or medically qualified Registrar. Very occasionally we have come across junior trainees who describes themselves as the 'Max-facs' doctors and, full of their imagined importance, attempt to deal with all matters that come to their attention; this is potentially dangerous. The writers still shudder with stress at the thought of the trainee who once supervised the deterioration of a patient with respiratory complications overnight without involving her seniors. Most OMFS junior trainees keep the boss informed of any complications they become aware of, either as a result of their own direct observation or more commonly by being informed by the nursing staff.

The patients most at risk of developing systemic complications after surgery are the elderly and medically unfit such as those who have pre-existing cardiovascular or respiratory disease or are immunocompromised, such as diabetics. The risks are increased for those having major surgery, cancer, reduced mobility or whose discharge from hospital is delayed for any number of reasons.

Most of the patients we operate on in the speciality of OMFS are medically fit and benefit from routine elective and non-urgent surgery. They can be assessed and their medical status optimised to reduce the risk of complications. Furthermore their stay in hospital is frequently brief; even patients having routine orthognathic surgery or fixation of facial fractures may be admitted for only one or two nights. The obvious exceptions to these are those with poly-trauma with facial injury; their stay in hospital is often prolonged by their other injuries. The patients we treat who are most likely to develop complications are those receiving surgery for cancer.

<u>Respiratory Complications</u>

Smokers and those with pre-existing Chronic Obstructive Pulmonary Disease (COPD) are those who are at greatest risk of respiratory complications; generally speaking anaesthetists are able to deal well with those with asthma.

During anaesthesia there is a decrease in action of the cilia lining the respiratory tract causing a decrease in clearance of secretions. This combined with the inability to cough and a decrease in ventilation will lead to an accumulation of secretions which may cause some obstruction and collapse of the peripheral airways called atelectasis. Atelectasis is most usually apparent as early and transient mild pyrexia; it usually resolves. Resolution is aided by early mobilisation, breathing exercises and, if necessary, chest physiotherapy to clear mucous accumulation; nebulised bronchodilators may help. Resolution is compromised by the cigarette smoking, COPD, obesity and immobility.

If atelectasis does not resolve adequately then the mucus accumulation will pre-dispose to secondary infection, often with nosocomial (hospital) organisms i.e. pneumonia. The signs and symptoms may include pyrexia, cough, discoloured sputum on coughing, chest pain on breathing (pleuritic), tachypnoea, a dull note on percussion of the affected part of the chest accompanied by reduced breath sounds on auscultation of that part. Treatment may involve physiotherapy and breathing exercises, oxygen, and antibiotics against organisms cultured from the sputum. In severe cases the patient may need ventilation.

A potential respiratory complication of OMFS is

Signs of Respiratory Complications

Pyrexia
Dyspnoea
Tachypnoea
Altered chest sounds

aspiration. The reason we see it so infrequently is because we take such care to avoid it. When operating on an anesthetised patient the anaesthetist uses a cuffed endo-tracheal tube or laryngeal mask airway to prevent aspiration of saliva, blood, tooth or bone fragments etc. and we pack off the pharynx and use suction for the same purpose. Patients are only anaesthetised if they have been starved to reduce the risk of aspiration of stomach contents into the lungs; in an emergency a naso-gastric tube will be passed by the anaesthetist to suction out stomach contents. Gastric acid can cause a chemical pneumonitis if it contaminates the lungs which can produce a secondary infection and pneumonia.

Cardiovascular Complications

You may be called by a ward nurse to tell you that a patient has post-operative hypotension. This should be reported to your superior; some of the causes may be serious but equally it can be benign. Patients may have a slightly low blood pressure as a result of medication such as ß-blockers or opiate analgesics given for pain. They may be slightly low on fluids and respond to having the end of the bed raised slightly or given some additional intra-venous fluid.

However it is necessary to consider that the patient has shock which is the term for inadequate tissue perfusion and oxygenation leading to cellular damage and organ dysfunction. This is serious.

Hypovolemic shock, where there has been a large blood loss, is an unusual complication in our speciality, although it must be considered. It is unlikely that a large blood loss would go unnoticed as we are usually operating within the mouth and blood loss will be noticed at the time. The patients must be assessed as a whole, particularly as young and fit patients have a high 'cardio-vascular reserve' and can compensate for a large blood loss before their pulse rate increases and blood pressure drops from loss of blood. Other signs of shock should be looked for, which include a cold clammy skin and poor capillary refill when squeezing

an extremity. Shock will also produce a decrease in core body temperature, decreased urinary output and in the case of hypovolemic shock a decreased central venous pressure. All these are measured during major cancer surgery to monitor the consequence of blood loss.

The management of hypovolemic shock will be to resuscitate with intravenous Hartmann's solution and find and arrest the bleeding. In the unlikely event you are first on the scene you should 'peek and shriek' i.e. you should rapidly assess the situation and call for help. In most cases the ward nurse will have realised the situation and already informed the intensive care out-reach team or the medical emergency team depending on the arrangements in your hospital.

Shock may be caused by inadequate cardiac output: cardiogenic shock. This may be caused by a myocardial infarct (MI), cardiac arrhythmias or left ventricular failure (LVF) as a consequence of coronary artery disease, previous MI or in elderly patients just from fluid overload. In most cases the patient will be elderly, have a cardiac history and be taking cardiac medication. The patient should be assessed by examination of the cardiovascular system looking for the signs of shock and ventricular failure. An ECG should be carried out and bloods tested for cardiac enzymes. This is a job for the medical emergency team or emergency physician on duty.

Occasionally you will see shock in an anaphylactic reaction; this should be managed as in the medical emergency chapter with the medical emergency team being called as necessary.

Deep vein thrombosis (DVT) within the deep veins of the legs is a particular later complication of surgery that you should know about and hopefully will never see as it is largely avoided though careful planning and prevention. After surgery there may be a slight hypercoagulability which may lead to a thrombosis in the deep veins of the leg. It is pre-disposed by immobility. Patients who are elderly, have cancer and

Signs of Cardio-Vascular Complications

Chest pain
Dyspnoea
Tachycardia
Confusion
Ankle swelling

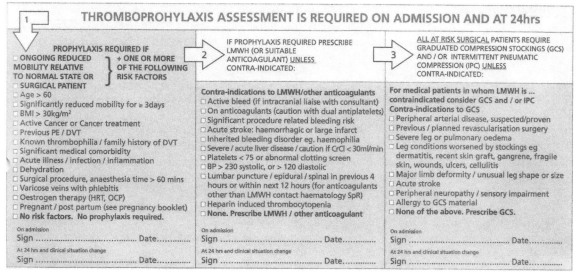

THROMBOPROHYLAXIS ASSESSMENT IS REQUIRED ON ADMISSION AND AT 24hrs

1	2	3
PROPHYLAXIS REQUIRED IF ☐ ONGOING REDUCED MOBILITY RELATIVE TO NORMAL STATE OR SURGICAL PATIENT + ONE OR MORE OF THE FOLLOWING RISK FACTORS	IF PROPHYLAXIS REQUIRED PRESCRIBE LMWH (OR SUITABLE ANTICOAGULANT) <u>UNLESS</u> CONTRA-INDICATED:	ALL AT RISK SURGICAL PATIENTS REQUIRE GRADUATED COMPRESSION STOCKINGS (GCS) AND / OR INTERMITTENT PNEUMATIC COMPRESSION (IPC) <u>UNLESS</u> CONTRA-INDICATED:
☐ Age > 60 ☐ Significantly reduced mobility for ≥ 3days ☐ BMI > 30kg/m² ☐ Active Cancer or Cancer treatment ☐ Previous PE / DVT ☐ Known thrombophilia / family history of DVT ☐ Significant medical comorbidity ☐ Acute illness / infection / inflammation ☐ Dehydration ☐ Surgical procedure, anaesthesia time > 60 mins ☐ Varicose veins with phlebitis ☐ Oestrogen therapy (HRT, OCP) ☐ Pregnant / post partum (see pregnancy booklet) ☐ **No risk factors. No prophylaxis required.**	**Contra-indications to LMWH/other anticoagulants** ☐ Active bleed (if intracranial liaise with consultant) ☐ On anticoagulants (caution with dual antiplatelets) ☐ Significant procedure related bleeding risk ☐ Acute stroke: haemorrhagic or large infarct ☐ Inherited bleeding disorder eg. haemophilia ☐ Severe / acute liver disease / caution if CrCl < 30ml/min ☐ Platelets < 75 or abnormal clotting screen ☐ BP > 230 systolic, or > 120 diastolic ☐ Lumbar puncture / epidural / spinal in previous 4 hours or within next 12 hours (for anticoagulants other than LMWH contact haematology SpR) ☐ Heparin induced thrombocytopenia ☐ **None. Prescribe LMWH / other anticoagulant**	**For medical patients in whom LMWH is ... contraindicated consider GCS and / or IPC** **Contra-indications to GCS** ☐ Peripheral arterial disease, suspected/proven ☐ Previous / planned revascularisation surgery ☐ Severe leg or pulmonary oedema ☐ Leg conditions worsened by stockings eg dermatitis, recent skin graft, gangrene, fragile skin, wounds, ulcers, cellulitis ☐ Major limb deformity / unusual leg shape or size ☐ Acute stroke ☐ Peripheral neuropathy / sensory impairment ☐ Allergy to GCS material ☐ **None of the above. Prescribe GCS.**
On admission Sign .... Date............. At 24 hrs and clinical situation change Sign .... Date..............	On admission Sign .... Date............. At 24 hrs and clinical situation change Sign .... Date..............	On admission Sign .... Date............. At 24 hrs and clinical situation change Sign .... Date..............

Thromboprohylaxis assessment form

have received major surgery are particularly at risk. The consequence may be varicose veins but more particularly a breaking off of the clot to produce an embolus in the lung leading to right sided heart failure and death. Prevention starts at the pre-operative assessment where all patients are considered for their risk. All hospitals have a thrombo-prophylaxis assessment check list form used for all patients who are admitted and receive general anaesthesia. You will be involved in completing these either electronically or manually.

Pneumatic compression of the calves during the operation prevents stasis within the veins of the legs. Thrombo-embolic deterrent (TED) stockings are worn by the patient while in hospital and low molecular weight heparin given after surgery to reduce the risk of clotting. You should be aware of the risks of the individual patients on the wards with whose care you are assisting and double check that they are getting the DVT prophylaxis they need.

DVT is usually silent with no physical signs but there may be an oedematous swelling of the affected leg or pyrexia; this usually occurs 5 -7 days after surgery. A pulmonary embolus may present as chest pain, shortness of breath, tachypnoea, acute right sided heart failure or sudden death.

Urinary Complications

The principal urinary problems that you are likely to come across in OMFS patients are decreased urinary output (oliguria), urinary tract infection and urinary retention.

Most of our patients are medically fit with normal renal function so the most likely cause of oliguria is that the patient has decreased output consequent upon inadequate fluid intake. In many of our major cases, particularly the long cancer cases which may involve significant blood loss, a urinary catheter will be placed in the operating theatre before surgery. Apart from the convenience of collecting urine when the patient is unconscious during surgery or in the post-operative period it allows the output to be measured which will help in calculating the fluid balance during surgery and beyond. Back on the ward one would normally expect a normal patient to produce 1.5 litres of urine a day i.e. about 60 mls. per hour; this will vary slightly. If several hours go by during which significantly less urine is produced then something is wrong and in the

Enoxaparin (Clexane). 40 mg in a pre-filled syringe is a low molecular weight heparin usually given subcutaneously after surgery to help prevent DVT

Deep Vein Thrombosis Prevention

Pneumatic compression stockings
TED stockings
Low molecular weight heparin
Mobilise early

Causes of Confusion
Hypoxia
Trauma
Drugs
Sepsis
Pain
Electrolyte imbalance
Dementia
Alcohol withdrawal

surgery. The causes of confusion are many; these include hypoxia, trauma, medication, sepsis, pain, dementia, electrolyte imbalance and alcohol withdrawal.

A full physical examination should be carried out to exclude hypoxia or sepsis and a review made of all the medication that the patient is taking. A new or recent full blood count and biochemistry profile should be considered for a significant decrease in haemoglobin or change in electrolyte balance. Pain control should be reviewed and medication adjusted to get optimal relief.

absence of renal disease it is most likely that they are 'dry' and need additional fluid.

Where there is complete obstruction of urine output then the urine will build up in the bladder and eventually the patient will be in pain and be distressed. The bladder will be distended and easily palpable above the pubis as a supra-pubic mass, palpation or pressure will be acutely uncomfortable or painful. If the patient has a catheter then it will be blocked and should be flushed with saline or replaced. The most likely cause, however, will be benign hypertrophy of the prostate gland which occurs commonly in elderly men. The patient will give a history of 'prostatic' symptoms indicating pre-existing outflow obstruction. These will include a poor stream on passing urine, hesitancy - delay in starting to micturate, dribbling - urine still leaking after stopping micturition and a feeling that the bladder has not properly emptied after micturition. The patient with urinary retention will be pleased to have a urinary catheter passed as this will give immediate relief of the pain and discomfort. They should then be referred to a urologist.

Patients should have had their alcohol intake considered at their pre-operative assessment. Those who have a very high intake and who are deprived for several days can become very confused and disorientated with both auditory and visual hallucinations; this can be very distressing for all concerned. The problem can be prevented by administering a small but regular amount of alcohol to the patient in the form of a few mls. of whisky if necessary through a gastrostomy or naso-gastric tube.

Most frequently confusion will be in an elderly patient with pre-existing dementia. Often an elderly patient will manage quite normally at home in their own environment but when admitted to hospital to an unusual noisy environment and then given additional medication and some pain they may become completely disorientated, confused, uncooperative and uncontrollable. In these cases assessment and management is best referred to a care of the elderly physician.

Urinary catheters should be removed as soon as possible after their function is no longer needed; otherwise they will act as a portal of infection into the urethra and bladder leading to discomfort and pyrexia. Where patients have had them inserted in theatre for major cancer cases they should be removed within a couple of days after surgery or as soon as measurement of urinary output is not needed. They should not be left in for the convenience of not having to help the patient to the bathroom. Apart from facilitating infection a catheter will predispose to ulceration of the lining of the urethra and adhesions leading to permanent urinary outflow obstruction. Patients' mobility is usually reduced by the presence and discomfort of a urinary catheter.

Post-Operative Confusion

Occasionally a patient may become confused after

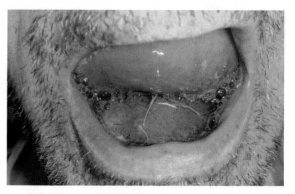

A radial forearm flap which has failed because the venous outflow has blocked. The patient will develop a severe pyrexia until the dead tissue is removed

Causes of Pyrexia

Early

 Atelectasis
Blood transfusion

Intermediate

 Infected catheters or lines
Tissue death
Chest infection

Late

 All the above
Surgical wound infection
Venous thrombosis

Pyrexia

All hospital inpatients have their temperature recorded regularly. Temperature can be measured in several ways e.g. oral, rectal, vaginal. In the operating theatre during our major cancer cases it is now usually measured within the bladder by a probe attached to a urinary catheter or by inserting a flexible rectal probe. On the ward, however, the most popular way is tympanic temperature using a probe placed into an ear; this is both quick and hygienic.

Normally temperature will vary at different times of the day, menstrual cycle, ambient room temperature, clothing and after food or drink. It is therefore not the absolute temperature we are concerned about as much as the variation in the particular patient. The temperature will vary around 37.5°C.

In the immediate post-operative period the most common causes of pyrexia will be atelectasis, as discussed above, or blood transfusion. Transfused blood is always matched for compatibility with the ABO and Rhesus systems. However there will be other antibodies which will cause a reaction in the host and hence a mild pyrexia.

In the intermediate period 3 to 5 days post-op a pyrexia is likely to be caused by infection particularly of in-dwelling catheters such as urinary catheters, central venous lines, peripheral venous lines etc. If the patient develops a wound infection at the site of operation it is unlikely to have developed enough to cause a rise in temperature by this stage. However frank tissue death such as a tissue flap used to reconstruct a

defect caused during cancer resection may well cause pyrexia if it is starting to lose vitality. You should check all the sites of lines and catheters for signs of inflammation, the operation site and report the pyrexia and your findings for your superior to review. You should also examine the chest in case atelectasis is developing into a chest infection.

A late pyrexia may be due to any of the above causes but in addition an infection at the operative site must be more seriously considered together with venous thrombosis.

Recognition of critical illness

In addition to recognising complications it is desirable that you should understand how to recognise someone who is 'going off' after surgery, i.e. becoming critically ill. However it is likely to be the ward nurse who raises the alarm. The nurse may alert the Intensive Care outreach team who will send one of their specialist nurses to assess the problem. The system will

Track & Trigger Scoring

Score	3	2	1	0	1	2	3
Temperature		<35		35-38.4		≥38.5	
Heart Rate		≤40	41-50	51-100	101-110	111-129	≥130
Systolic BP	<70	71-80	81-100	101-199		>200	
Respiratory Rate		<9		9-16	17-20	21-29	≥30
Oxygen saturation	<85	85-89	90-94	≥95			
Conscious level			New Agitation / Confusion	Alert	Voice	Pain	Unresponsive

	Score	Alert
	0-1	• Observations 6-12 hourly
Low	2-3	• Patient has potential to deteriorate • Increase observations to a minimum of 2-4 hourly • Alert the nurse in charge • Requires extra vigilance
Medium	4-6	• Patient is acutely unwell • Urgent call to the patient team • Assess patient and increase observations to at least 1 hourly • Use Track & Trigger Step Up Chart • Ensure effective management plan is developed • Contact Outreach / Hospital at night for review
High	7 or more	• Patient is critically unwell • Emergency call to patient team and senior staff • Assess patient / Hospital at night as soon as • Continue observations as Track & Trigger Step Up Chart • Continuous monitoring
	What if DNAR or escalation inappropriate?	• Continue close observations • Contact own team for review • Contact outreach team for advice

Do not hesitate to contact the Medical Emergency Team/ Cardiac Arrest team if patient has collapsed, is rapidly deteriorating or you have major concerns DIAL 2222

Medical Early Warning Score sheet. Based on the patient's observation charts, these are used by the ward nurses to indicate when to call for help when a patient is deteriorating.

be different between hospitals; in some it may the medical emergency team who is alerted; in others it may be you who is called, in which case you should make a brief assessment but not delay passing the problem up the chain of command.

The onset of complications can often be followed by the nurses' observation charts which will be kept in the patient's nursing folder at the end of the bed. You should learn to be familiar with these which normally record the patient's pulse rate, blood pressure, respiratory rate and temperature. After major surgery, such as a head and neck cancer resection and reconstruction, the patient will also have oxygen saturation monitoring, a fluid input and output chart; urine output measurement will be possible because of a urinary catheter.

The onset of problems must be suspected if the patient's temperature or pulse rate is consistently raised or their oxygen saturation decreases. Decrease in blood pressure is often a late change in hypovolaemia due to physiological compensation; it should always be treated seriously. A decrease in urine output is potentially a bad sign.

The most significant observational signs in terms of indicating critical illness are the respiratory rate and pulse with blood pressure. The normal respiratory rate should be between 12 and 20 per minute. If this rate is higher than this or is increasing this is a significant indication that all is not well. If the pulse rate is above the systolic blood pressure this too is serious and requires immediate medical attention. This is known as the 'Portsmouth' sign.

17. <u>Understanding the Intensive Care Unit</u>

The Intensive Care Unit (ICU) provides a higher level of monitoring and support for seriously ill or deteriorating patients than is available on the general wards. This will include mechanical ventilation and complex support for patients with multiple organ failure. In practice, most patients on ICU have cardiovascular or respiratory problems, electrolyte and renal malfunction, or depressed consciousness. In many cases this may have been triggered or exacerbated by sepsis of one sort or another.

ICU also provides an outreach service to advise about patients on the wards who have a physiological abnormality which is at risk of deteriorating. The intention is to help reverse this and avoid an Intensive Care admission. Patients may be referred directly to the ICU outreach service by ward nurses. This will be triggered by a scoring system based on a chart called the Modified Early Warning System, which has been shown to be an accurate predictor of clinical deterioration (see previous chapter). Patients receive intensive care only if they are likely to benefit from it, not just because they are seriously ill; they will not benefit from it if death from their presenting condition is inevitable, for example uncontrolled cancer or end stage cardiac failure.

Admission to ICU may be from the Accident and Emergency Department, from the general wards, or from the operating theatre. Some patients may be booked into ICU in advance if they are having major surgery and they have serious co-morbidity such as cardiac or respiratory disease.

On 'the unit', patients are looked after by the specialist 'intensivists' who are usually specialist

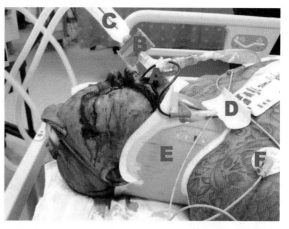

A patient admitted to ICU 3 hours after a motorcycle accident. His only injuries were a fractured arm and maxilla. He has been heavily sedated with Propofol and is being artificially ventilated through an oral endotrachael tube because of massive facial swelling which would otherwise obstruct his airway. A. endotrachael tube B. air filter C. breathing circuit to ventilator D. bag attached to gastric tube to aspirate stomach contents to prevent regurgitation E. rigid neck collar to stabilize cervical spine (all patients with severe facial injuries are assumed to have cervical spine injuries until they have been X rayed or CT scanned and cleared by an orthopaedic surgeon) F. ECG electrode. I operated on him a week later & he was discharged home 2 days after that.

anaesthetists. They are assisted by a large team of other professionals, most numerous of whom are the specialist ITU nurses. Each patient will have a nurse solely assigned to them. Where surgeons are involved with the patients there will be shared care; the surgical team should visit each day to contribute advice from the surgical perspective. All treatment orders and prescriptions requested by the surgeons should be formally written by the intensivists; this avoids any confusion.

Patients who require Oral and Maxillofacial Surgery care shared with Intensive Care usually fall mostly within two categories. Firstly, patients who are receiving major resections of cancers of the head and neck, often with soft tissue flap repair, and secondly, patients with multiple injuries which include face and jaw injury. Occasionally we may have a patient in the

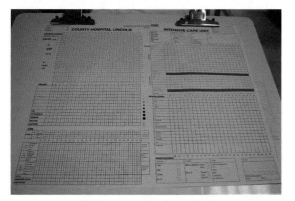

Patient monitoring chart

ICU who has major oro-facial sepsis, usually caused by a dental abscess.

Most patients having major head and neck cancer resection will be transferred from the recovery unit in theatres directly to the ward for post operative care. However they may go to ITU if they have co-existing severe cardiac or respiratory disease, especially where post operative ventilation is desirable. Similarly, most patients with facial injuries will not need intensive care as facial injuries are not life threatening unless there is severe bleeding or airways obstruction. However, patients with multiple injuries, particularly of the head or chest, may need intensive care. The facial injuries are usually dealt with when the life threatening injuries have been stabilised; the Maxillofacial team will have to liaise with the intensivists over the best time to operate.

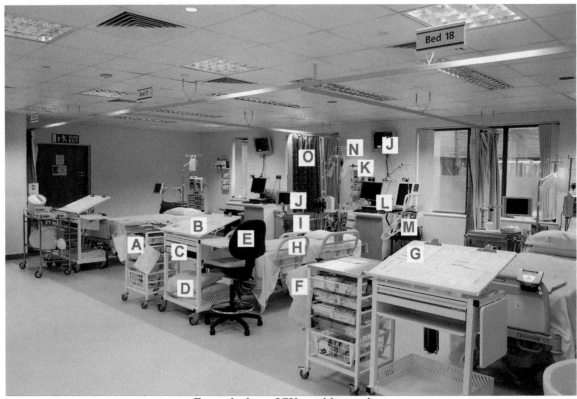

Empty beds on ICU awaiting patients

A. Trolley containing trays of small equipment. Syringes, needles, specimen bottles, gloves, microbiology swabs etc.
B. Monitoring charts
C. ICU & hospital notes in loose leaf folder
D. Spare pillows
E. Stool for nurse
F. Waste bags. Yellow for clinical waste, black (hidden) for non clinical and rigid yellow sharps bin
G. Advice leaflet for relatives
H. Bed for patient
I. Monitoring equipment

J. Video monitor for ECG., blood pressure, PO_2, CO_2, temperature, venous pressure, airways gases and pressure
K. Disposable protective aprons (on wall) with 3 sizes of non sterile disposable gloves beneath
L. Hospital computer system
M. Ventilator
N. Drip stand for infusions
O. Curtain between beds for privacy

18. <u>Being On Call, Accidents and Emergencies</u>

Oral and Maxillofacial Surgery is a 24 hour speciality so you can expect patients with urgent conditions to present at any time during the day and night. In addition there will patients on the wards who may need attention at any time.

In some OMFS departments, which cover a large populated area, the work from the Accident and Emergency department (A&E) may be of such a volume that you may work a shift system. In others you may work normal hours and simply take your turn at being on-call in the evening or at night. The latter is preferable as you are there to learn what you can which will be useful to you in your future career in dentistry. If you are on a shift at night suturing facial lacerations and admitting patients with broken jaws you will not be able to be up in the morning and seeing patients in clinics and learning from them.

If you are up all night working a shift it is reasonable for you have to attend the wards to see patients that need night sedation written up or IV drips resited and other small tasks. If you are on-call you should not be asked to have to get up to deal with these things. There should be a 'hospital at night' team to deal with them which should include 'clinical support workers' who deal with IV drips and drugs.

The Accident and Emergency Department (A&E) exists to manage patients who have suffered accidents and emergencies, the definition in the medical sense of an emergency being 'a sudden or unexpected event which is potentially life threatening'. It therefore should not include toothache, broken teeth (unless resulting from an accident), complications of minor oral surgery or anybody with anything who finds it more convenient to attend out of normal working hours rather than to the outpatient clinic during the day.

A&E medicine is a speciality in its own right and the department will have its own Consultants and supporting staff who may be known as casualty officers. In good A&E departments the most junior trainees will be supported for most of the time by more senior doctors who will probably include a substantial contingent of associate specialists, staff grade surgeons and clinical assistants who will be general medical practitioners doing some sessional work within the hospital. Most A&E departments will have their own

ward to which the casualty doctors admit patients, usually just overnight, under their care. Patients referred to specialist services will usually be admitted to their own wards.

You should be very understanding of the A&E doctors as they have the worst job in the hospital, having to be Jacks of everybody's trade and having to have an understanding of every other speciality and when to manage or refer patients on. Your interaction with trainee doctors in A&E may be pivotal in their attitude to the OMFS speciality for the rest of their careers.

Although A&E will inevitably receive some patients with major multiple injuries, which will include facial injuries to be managed by the OMFS service, the majority of the work will be on the 'walking wounded'. These will include soft tissue lacerations from fights and falls, dental injuries, dog bites to the face (particularly in children), and facial fractures, mostly from interpersonal violence.

Patients will be seen initially by a triage nurse who will decide the priority of their problems and make initial notes. Patients with minor ailments may be given advice and sent on their way to see their GP the next day. After seeing the nurse the patients will either be seen by the casualty doctor and assessed by them or referred to specialist services if necessary; this may include you.

When you first encounter an injured patient, like all clinical encounters with patients, you should have an order in your mind as to how you are going to go about things. Traditionally doctors have relied on firstly taking a history before examining the patient and then ordering special tests. This still seems to be the safest way of proceeding. If you follow the sequence with clear headings in your mind you will reduce the risk of missing anything.

The history involves details about the injury, time and place and cause etc. and any 'complaints' the patient may have. Sometimes it is difficult to phrase the questioning. The inebriated patient with a battered and bruised face whose mandible is in three pieces does not respond amicably to being asked if it hurts. Some things are self-evident but certain "direct questions" have to be asked if not volunteered – loss of

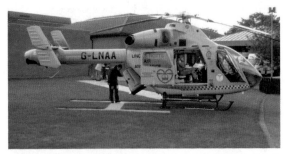

Although some patients will be brought in by ambulance and a few by ambucopter the majority you see will be walking wounded.

consciousness, the site of pain, associated facial numbness, abnormality of bite and when they last ate or drank. Needless to say you need a medical and social history and the former is no different from that which you would take from a dental patient. The latter concentrates on practical aspects of the patient's future care:- occupation, whether they live alone, whether they are accompanied by someone who can take them home when necessary.

You should document injuries by drawing bruising and lacerations, preferably with measurements, and make sure you check for facial numbness and facial movement before you treat the patient. Someone with a facial palsy following suturing under local anaesthetic may claim you caused it and after you have put the local anaesthetic in it is too late to check. Similarly you must record numbness of the lower lip or cheek before treatment of a fractured mandible or zygoma to ensure that the surgeon is not blamed for damaging the mandibular or infra-orbital nerve with his surgery.

Records written in the A&E department are those most likely to be referred to later, often for the purpose of insurance or legal claims or police statements. It is vitally important that your notes are legible and comprehensive. The date and time you saw the patient must be clearly written; this should include the year. It is very frustrating to return to records several months or years later to find the date has been missed out. It indicates carelessness.

There will be many occasions when you will be the first called upon to diagnose fractures of the facial skeleton. After a short while the common patterns of

injury will become obvious to you and the task will become easy. Except in a very few unusual cases of severe haemorrhage, bony facial injuries are not life threatening and can be dealt with at a leisurely pace. Most injuries will be to the mandible and zygoma. In many cases such as mandibular condyle or malar injuries, the patient can be discharged home with analgesics and asked to attend the outpatient clinic for assessment when the swelling has subsided and the occlusion and any cosmetic malar flattening can be more easily assessed. However, most patients with mandibular fractures will need to be admitted to hospital for operation, usually the following day. They should have a venous cannula placed and intra venous fluids and antibiotics started. If the patient has a very displaced mandibular fracture a bridle wire may be applied around teeth adjacent to the fracture to partly reduce it. This will help prevent movement and hence minimize pain and swelling.

Displaced teeth should be reduced and splinted as soon as possible using local anaesthetic and temporary splinting material. Our preferred method is to splint the teeth with thermoplastic special tray plastic as a temporary measure and then to bring the patient back to the outpatient clinic in working hours and make a splint using orthodontic brackets and wires attached using an acid etch technique. This allows the tooth some physiological movement and a reduced chance of ankylosis.

The A&E Department will probably not stock the instruments or keep the materials you will need to give first aid for dental injuries or to suture and pack bleeding extraction sockets. In our department we keep these in a toolbox which our surgeons can carry to A&E and which is kept stocked by our staff nurse. Most departments will have similar arrangements. We suggest you find out where you may find instruments and familiarize yourself with them before you see patients.

Some patients will present with multiple injuries. With the exception of airway obstruction or uncontrolled bleeding the facial injuries should be considered after those injuries which are potentially life threatening. The A&E doctor will have made an initial assessment. If the patient has soft tissue facial lacerations and/or loose or badly damaged teeth it may be appropriate to operate on these at the same time if the patient is being taken to the operating theatre for treatment of orthopaedic or abdominal injuries.

Definitive management of facial fractures is best deferred until better imaging and consent is obtained. The second on call should always be informed if a patient presents with facial injuries so that an appropriate assessment can be made, appropriate notes written and the management of the face planned in context with the other injuries that may be present.

When you have seen patients in A&E you will have to make a decision about follow up. When you start your first job you will need to contact the person second on call to you to see the patient or for verbal guidance. However, you will soon become confident about which patients should be admitted to a surgical ward and which can come back to an outpatient clinic for follow up or assessment. You will need to know in advance which are the best clinic days to bring patients back to so that you can tell them.

We repeat: clinical notes written in A&E are particularly important, not only because of the management of the patient but because they may be used in the preparation of police statements, compensation claims and for medical reports for personal injury insurance claims. It is necessary to write full details about the injuries sustained, with measurements of lacerations and a note of which teeth have been damaged and how much. You should make a note of the time you have seen the patient and print your name so that you are easily identified.

A special word about toothache. At some stage someone is going to call you for a patient who has

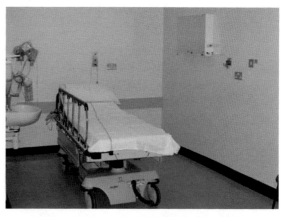

Most patients you will have to deal with will be presented to you on a trolley in a treatment cubicle. You should attempt to deal with the patient as swiftly as possible and if suturing is likely to be prolonged move them to the ward or outpatient clinic.

dental pain. There will always be some reason they cannot see a dentist in normal hours. Almost certainly you will not have the facilities to attend to them properly; in particular you will not have a drill and endodontic equipment to deal with pulpitis, or forceps and surgical kit to do extractions. There will be no materials to do dental dressings and there will be no nurse trained with dental procedures to chaperone and assist you. You will only be able to provide sympathy and Ibuprofen. The latter can be bought over the counter at a pharmacy or the 24 hour supermarket nearby.

If you do see patients with dental pain you will not only remove the responsibility from those who should organise a dental emergency service, it will be considered by local A&E staff that this is your raison d'être. If repeated elsewhere, a new generation of junior hospital doctors will evolve whose attitude to OMFS will have regressed to that prevalent 25 years ago – you will be the hospital dentist and soon you will be inundated.

Some trauma centres or OMFS departments will require you to input data after you have been on-call to the department's trauma database. This is not only helpful to the department and hospital but can also generate audit projects which all junior trainees need to do and demonstrate at their appraisal. This will help you tremendously when you apply for your next job in your career progression.

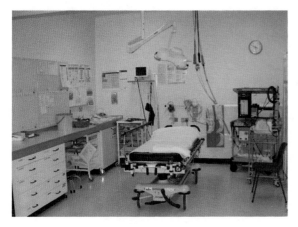

Those with serious injuries are brought from the ambulance on a trolley straight to the resuscitation room. This contains anaesthetic and other equipment for resuscitation.

19. <u>Wound Closure - Skin Suturing</u>

Possibly your most satisfying work will be attending to soft tissue lacerations. Our experience has been that our dentally qualified trainees have developed a manual dexterity at this stage of their career which makes them ideally suited to facial soft tissue work. In addition to this, the casualty doctors may not have sufficient time to produce an ideal result. Time is another main ingredient for a nice cosmetic result. At first you will be uncertain of yourself but you will soon master the techniques and be producing rewarding results. Try to arrange for patients you have treated to be reviewed in an outpatient clinic at a time when you will be able to have the satisfaction of seeing the results of your good work.

In general terms the best time to close facial lacerations is immediately, using local analgesia in the A&E department, although severe, multiple and complex soft tissue injuries may need a general anaesthetic for the best cosmetic result. If the procedure is going to be prolonged, i.e. more than half an hour, we would consider transferring the patient to another facility, for example, the OMFS outpatient clinic during the working day or the ward at night; facilities and accepted procedures will vary between different hospitals. It may well be difficult to spend an hour or more producing a nice cosmetic result with a nurse assisting you when all in the A&E department is bedlam, with a serious injury in the resuscitation room and the corridor stacked with trolleys of patients needing attention. In these circumstances it may be better to dress the wounds and admit the patient to the ward and suture later in operating theatre, or the following morning.

We would have a lower threshold for postponing suturing of drunks. However, each case must be treated on its merits. While an amiable elderly drunk may snore away soundly while you suture his face, the treatment of a young aggressive lout may be better postponed until the following morning when he may be better able to cooperate for an improved result. Drunks are better admitted to the A&E ward overnight where they can be in the company of other inebriates rather than onto a surgical ward where they will be likely to be a nuisance to the God-fearing ill. Do not be tempted to admit the drunk with minor facial injuries under the care of OMFS only because the casualty doctor is reluctant to discharge them. If the

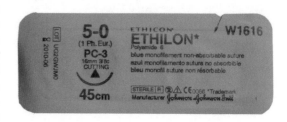

Polyamide (Nylon) trade name Ethilon. This is monofilament, i.e. it is not braided and therefore cleaner and excites very little local inflammation. It is therefore suitable for a good cosmetic result on the face but needs to be removed in 5 to 7 days. It is strong but brittle and can easily break when it is being tied. The material retains a memory so the knots can easily come undone so you need to pace 2 throws in both directions. Use 5-0 (which is very fine) for most areas of the face where a good cosmetic result is needed, and use 4-0 elsewhere such as the neck.

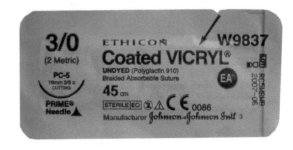

Untreated Polyglactin (Vicryl) is stronger, dissolves more slowly and is easier to handle as it is less fragile and likely to break. We would use it where we want the wound to be stronger and watertight as for orthognathic or cancer surgery or just for strength as when putting deep sutures in the scalp. It is coated with a copolymer of lactide and glycolide which slows loss of tensile strength and promotes more rapid absorption when the strength is lost. It is also coated with calcium stearate, which helps with tissue passage and smoothness of the knot tie.

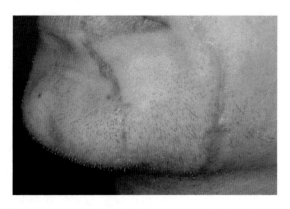

Dirt tattoo caused by inadequate wound cleaning before suturing

although it needs to be removed, gives a much better cosmetic result. Sometimes an uncooperative child may need a second anaesthetic five days later for removal of nylon sutures; this will usually be better than compromising a good aesthetic result by placing absorbable sutures which may leave point scars on the skin. We never use fibrin glue to close wounds on children as the final result is usually inferior to nylon sutures or synthetic monofilament resorbable sutures such as Monocryl.

facial injury does not require admission then the patient does not require admission under OMFS. Similarly if the patient has another serious injury, such as to the head or chest, they should not be admitted under our care.

Children require special consideration, rather than any special skill, in the management of their soft tissue injuries. In most cases the injuries will result from falls or dog bites. The former technique of wrapping a small child in a blanket and suturing (badly) with local anaesthetic while the child struggles is to be abhorred. A small child should be admitted to the children's ward, the paediatrician informed and arrangements made for a paediatric anaesthetist to administer the following morning. This should preferably be the first case on an emergency operating list so that the child is not starved for a long period. In the case of some small wounds it will be acceptable for a dressing to be put in place and the child to go home with the parents and return first thing in the morning. Some hospitals, particularly if they have a dedicated paediatric A&E department may provide a dedicated anaesthetist who may give a ketamine anaesthetic to allow closure of facial wounds without the need for the child to be admitted to a ward.

For children we always obtain consent for "examination under anaesthesia, clean and repair wounds as necessary". It is much better not to distress the child and parents with a detailed and uncomfortable deep examination of a wound and intra oral examination when all will be revealed more easily later under general anaesthesia. You may resist the temptation to place absorbable sutures through the epidermis of the skin rather than nylon which,

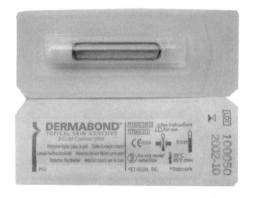

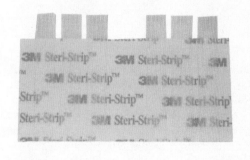

Cyanoacrylate glue (Dermobond) and adhesive tape (Steri-Strip) can be used as a temporary measure or as a definitive closure for a previously battle scarred uncooperative drunk. Tape can be used for very superficial cuts or to augment the strength of a sutured wound. Resist the temptation to use either as a definitive treatment for a small, tired and fractious child who is uncooperative. The glue will give a less than ideal tissue closure with a sub optimal cosmetic result and the child will have the strips off before they get to the bus stop. Get them back the next day and suture properly with a GA, even if it means a second anaesthetic for suture removal. Mother will want the very best result.

As with all practical tasks you should acclimatise yourself to the instruments and materials before you first approach a patient, and get the feel of them by practising on a suturing manikin. We preferentially use pig skin for this purpose as it allows the dermis and epidermis to be closed separately, although the layers are not so easily defined as in human skin which is therefore easier to sew.

You should initially examine the patient, ensure that there are no other facial or dental injuries and record the injuries in the notes. If the wound is deep or penetrating underlying structures such as the facial nerve, parotid duct or alar nasal cartilages may be involved; in these cases you should get help from your superiors.

Where tissue is missing it may be better to allow that part to heal by secondary intention rather than stretch the skin which may result in unsightly contractions later. This is particularly so around the eye; tension of skin may lead to ectropion (distortion of the lower eyelid pulled away from the conjunctiva), which is unsightly. For sewing wounds of the eyelid consult with an oculoplastic surgeon, if one can be found and persuaded to be interested.

Reassure the patient, make sure your assistant has the correct instruments ready, ensure the patient is in a comfortable position, that there are adequate surgical drapes in place and that you have a good operating light. You should then apply local anaesthetic. We use lignocaine and adrenaline from dental cartridges because the dental needles are so fine. The wound should be thoroughly cleaned with surgical swabs and sterile saline, ensuring any road dirt is scrubbed from the wounds and any grazed skin; otherwise it may produce unsightly skin tattooing. Any blood clot should be completely removed; the wound edges should be rubbed clean until fresh bleeding occurs.

The wound should then be closed with sutures. If it is deep, any dead space should be closed with 4/0 treated polyglactin (Vicryl rapide), using the minimum number of sutures. Following this the dermis should be closed using the same material with the knots buried away from the surface. Finally the epidermis should be closed with 5/0 or 4/0 Polypropylene (Prolene) or Nylon (Ethilon). The main mistake made by new surgeons is to place too many sutures; every suture is a foreign body which can promote infection, and deep absorbable sutures can lead to stitch abscesses. Always use just the minimum needed to neatly oppose the skin edges.

Generally speaking patients with facial lacerations should not be given antibiotics. This policy may be varied if the patient has particularly deep contaminated wounds or other associated compound bony injury. The A&E nurse will normally check the patients tetanus immunisation status and give a booster if required. Facial skin wounds are usually better without dressings, especially adherent ones. Chloramphenicol cream applied to the wound twice daily by the patient may help reduce secondary infection and prevent scab formation; this will make suture removal easier.

Arrangements should be made with the patient for the sutures to be removed either by the GP's nurse or in the outpatient department, depending upon convenience, the patient's wishes and local policy; this is best done in about 5 days for facial skin. The patients should be advised that non-absorbable sutures are used in the surface of the skin as they produce a better cosmetic result than dissolvable ones. However, if you are suturing the scalp within the hair line this will not matter.

Key Points

- Close simple facial lacerations immediately after debridement under local anaesthesia

- For complex wounds requiring general anaesthesia – dress the wound, admit to ward and contact 2nd on call

- Missing soft tissue, deep and penetrating injuries involving special underlying structures – get help from your supervisor

- Thorough debridement of any contaminated wounds (e.g. road dirt) to avoid unsightly skin tattooing

- Remove blood clots for examination and rub wound edges clean for fresh bleeding

- Antibiotics for deep contaminated wounds and compound bony injury

- Tetanus toxoid booster after checking immunisation status

- Removal of facial sutures in about 5 days by GP's nurse or OMFS outpatient department

How to describe a suture

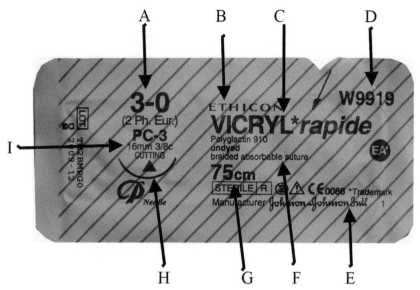

A B C D

I

H G F E

A: *The USP (United States Pharmacopeia) size definition of the thread diameter. You will only use 3/0 (0.2mm diam.) 4-0 (.015 mm diam.) or 5-0 (0.1 mm diam). The larger the number the finer the thread. Use 4-0 for deep sutures in the face unless the wound is on the scalp, in which case you will need something much stronger.* **B**: *The manufacturer.* **C**: *The trade name for the suture.* **D**: *The number for the individual suture.* **E**: *The parent company* **F**: *The material the suture is made of, its filament type and whether it is absorbable.* **G**: *The length of the thread.* **H**: *Diagram of the needle shape, laterally and in cross section. Needles may be straight or curved, cutting or round bodied. You will use exclusively curved cutting needles* **I**: *Description of the needle in words*

Polyglactin braided absorbable suture material (Vicryl) is the most commonly used in our department. There is Vicryl rapide which means that it is Vicryl which has been treated with gamma rays to increase the speed of absorption. It dissolves fairly quickly but gives only minimal support and is ideal for dento-alveolar surgery where soft tissue flap support is needed for only a few days. It is also used for deep sutures beneath the skin surface which likewise need only minimal support and quick absorption is an advantage. It is only fair in handling quality, being fairly brittle; it will easily break if you pull too tightly when tying. However, it knots fairly well; the knots tend to be stable and don't loosen.

So if you want this suture (which you frequently will) you would ask the nurse for a '3/0 Vicryl rapide on a curved cutting needle please.' You will then probably be shown the unopened packet so that you can look at, and approve, the needle size rather like a

waiter shows you the label on a bottle of wine. Alternately, if you can remember it, you can just ask for the suture number : 'a W9919 please.'

How to place a skin suture

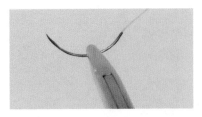

1. Hold the suture needle in the centre at 90 degrees. Try not to deviate from this position; you will find it difficult at first but in time this practice will pay off.

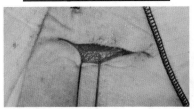

2. Before closing a traumatic wound ensure that it is clean by washing with surgical swabs soaked in saline. Close any deep tissue space with minimal deep sutures. Avoid causing unnecessary trauma to the skin with the forceps.

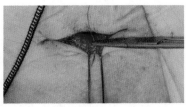

3. First place a suture through the dermis from below upwards; the aim is to bury the knot away from the skin surface. Hold the skin margin closest to you and pass a Vicryl suture needle towards you through the dermal layer.

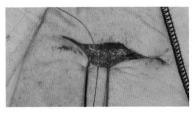

4. and pull the suture through towards you.

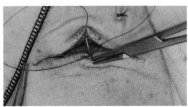

5. Now do the opposite. Pass the needle through the dermis furthest away from you, from above down and pull it through towards you.

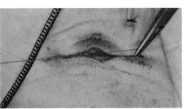

6. Tie the knot 2 throws one way & one the other. The knot should be buried with the knotted strands both the same side of the superficial strand of the loop.

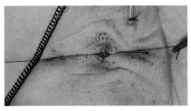

7' Tighten the knot and cut it short.

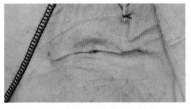

8. Place more sutures to close the rest of the dermis. Use minimal sutures; beginners usually place too many.

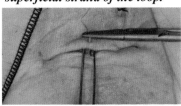

9. Pass a nylon suture through the epidermal layer furthest away from you from above down.

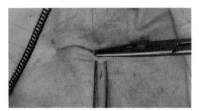

10. Then through the epidermis closest to you from below up.

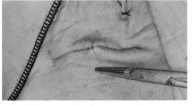

11. Tie the knot two throws one way, one the other and another two the first way as this material is inclined to slip and the suture needs an extra throw to secure it.

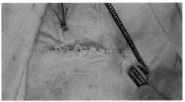

12. Apply chloramphenicol cream and give the patient a supply to take home to apply twice daily. Superficial sutures should be removed in 5 to 7 days on the face.

20. <u>Dealing with Bleeding from the Mouth</u>

Sometimes patients will present to the A&E Department with haemorrhage after dental extraction performed outside of the hospital. The patient may present to the hospital either of their own volition or because the dentist who carried out the extraction has not been contactable.

Patients who are bleeding must be seen and treated. Suturing the sockets and packing them with oxidised cellulose gauze is usually effective but sometimes haemorrhage can be persistent and require hospital admission.

When you arrive you will probably find that the patient is biting on a gauze swab or spitting blood and saliva into a kidney bowl they have been given for the purpose; the bowl may contain many blood stained swabs and the patient may be distressed.

At first you should sit the patient comfortably and not quite horizontal on a treatment trolley with a good light and suction. Decontaminate your hands and place on personal protective equipment and gloves. Suck out the patient's mouth to observe where the bleeding is coming from and get them to bite on a tightly folded swab for 15 minutes.

You should then take a full history which should include how long they have been bleeding for, where the surgery was carried out and what was done, whether they were given any instructions, if they have been rinsing their mouth etc. A medical history is mandatory including any previous surgery and associated bleeding, bruising or abnormal bleeding if they cut themselves. Enquire about their medical status. Bleeding can result from liver disease caused by alcohol abuse, hepatitis or cancer, bone marrow disease from cancer, such as leukaemia or recent cancer chemotherapy. Platelet function can be compromised by renal disease or auto-immune thrombocytopenia.

There are many drugs which may contribute towards haemorrhage including aspirin and dipyridamole. If the patient is taking the anti-coagulant warfarin its action may be potentiated by other medications such as anti-hypertensives, antifungals, carbamazepine, steroids, phenytoin, aspirin, and antibiotics such as erythromycin and metronidazole.

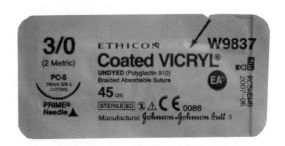

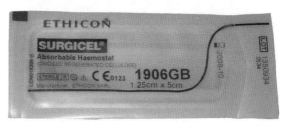

Bleeding after dental extraction is usually stopped by pressure from biting on a gauze swab for 20 minutes followed by packing the socket with oxidized cellulose gauze (Surgicel) and suturing with 3/0 Vicryl. Tranexamic acid given intravenously is wonderful for difficult cases.

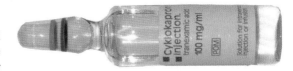

If warfarin is being used a blood sample should be taken to check the INR (International Normalised Ratio - see later chapter on haematology tests). Even if the ratio is higher than it should be bleeding can usually be stopped with local measures without the need to reverse the warfarin with vitamin K. Very occasionally reversal will be needed. A haematologist should be called if the ratio is very high and bleeding cannot be stopped with local measures. Newer anti-coagulants, rivaroxaban and dabigatran, have no antidote but their effect can be diminished by stopping the medication as they have shorter half-lives.

Once the history has been taken and the patient has bitten on a swab for 15 minutes the situation can be re-assessed and local anaesthetic with vasoconstrictor can be infiltrated and the wound packed with oxidised surgical gauze and sutures with

Vicryl. In persistent cases a tranexamic acid mouthwash may also be helpful. Also 500 mgs of tranexamic acid may be given intravenously; this can be very helpful in stopping dental haemorrhage that does not respond to the simplest operative method, but it should be used with caution in the elderly or those with history of thrombosis.

A patient who has suffered from bleeding in this way should always have a routine full blood count and coagulation screen. Very few patients who present with bleeding in this way will have platelet or coagulation problems, but a significant number of patients who do have platelet or coagulation problems are initially diagnosed after a dental haemorrhage. These simple screening tests will be automatically reviewed by a haematologist and if abnormal will be investigated in more detail.

We have a low threshold for admitting the patient to hospital overnight, particularly if they are elderly, live some distance away or are distressed. Often a small dose of narcotic analgesia (i.e. morphine 5mgs. subcutaneously) in these circumstances will help settle them for the night and help relieve their anxiety.

Key Points

●Patients who are bleeding from sockets must be seen promptly – local anaesthetic with vasoconstrictor, pack with oxidised cellulose gauze, suture sockets, tranexamic acid mouth wash

●If persisted haemorrhage – requires hospital admission

●Identify source of bleeding by sucking out patient's mouth – bite on tightly folded swab

●Obtain full history and medical history

●Drugs contributing to haemorrhage – aspirin, dipyridamole, warfarin

●Warfarin can be potentiated by antihypertensives, antifungals, steroids, antibiotic. etc

●Check INR for patient on warfarin – seldom requires Vitamin K for reversal

●New anticoagulants – rivaroxaban and dabigatran – no antidote and have shorter half-life

---

21. <u>Examination of the Injured Face</u>

One of the tasks you will be expected to fulfil as a member of the OMFS team is to go to the Accident and Emergency Department to examine a patient with an injured face. This may appear daunting at first but should be quite simple if you are prepared. You should follow a sequence of steps in a methodical manner, making notes as you go. After about half a dozen patients it will be easy, and soon after that it should be as easy as measuring periodontal pockets.

You will also need to look at facial images, either X-rays or CT scans. These may initially appear to be complicated, but are also fairly simple if you approach it methodically (see next chapter). It goes without saying that someone more senior should also examine the patient before any decision is made about the need, or otherwise, for treatment. This need not necessarily be at the same time or visit to the hospital.

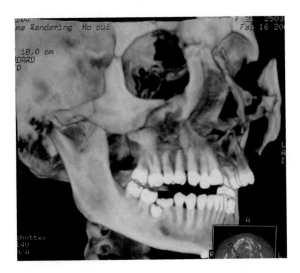

3-D CT scan of mid face fracture. This is almost as bad as it gets and could happen to you if you don't wear a seat belt.

Most of the trauma patients with suspected facial fractures will present at the Accident and Emergency Department as a result of interpersonal violence. Most will not have any other injuries but may have some facial cuts or abrasions, bruising and swelling. Patients with cuts will need to have them sutured; loosened or displaced teeth will need to be repositioned and splinted; patients with fractures of the mandible will probably need admitting to hospital for urgent (but not emergency) surgery. Some patients with facial trauma

will be able to go home again and return to an outpatient or dedicated trauma clinic a day or two later when the swelling has subsided for assessment by the Consultant.

Although most facial injuries, caused by falls or fights, are fairly minor there are also more severe injuries resulting from road accidents but these are much fewer due to seat belts and air bags. A few patients will have multiple injuries. By and large, facial injuries will usually wait until after life threatening injuries are dealt with. Fractures of the face are rarely a threat to life, whereas head, thorax, abdominal or limb injuries frequently are. Very occasionally you may be called to someone who is bleeding profusely from the face. Here you will need to make a very superficial and quick assessment of the situation and call the second on call, who will be a Specialist Registrar or Consultant.

In the assessment of facial trauma, diagnosis is 80% clinical examination and 20% imaging. Far too many X-rays are ordered in the Accident and Emergency Department, usually by the casualty officers, before you get called. Always get into the habit of examining the patient before looking at any X-rays and don't tell the patient they have a fracture unless you are absolutely sure. On many occasions we have examined trauma patients in the outpatient clinic who have been disappointed to learn that they have no fracture when they had been looking forward to a pay-out from the Criminal Injuries Compensation Authority and this is now denied them.

Before examining the face it is important to take a history and write good notes. The initial Accident and Emergency notes you write are those most likely to be read and used some time after the event, even years later. This is because they may be needed in the preparation of reports for solicitors, for compensation claims and statements for the police. It is possible that several years after you have moved from the job a legal argument over causation of an injury may depend upon the notes you have written, which should include a record of negative as well as positive findings.

We would always advise that you ask the patient about, and record evidence of, other injuries, even superficial bruises and abrasions as these may be of legal relevance at a later date. Ask the patient if they lost consciousness and whether they can remember the incident. This will be of relevance in assessing any degree of head injury but it is also worth recording for its own sake. We continue to be surprised over just how many of our clients cannot remember the incident in which their injury was caused but become quite lucid at a later date when a policeman or a friend explains that they may be able to make a compensation claim. Likewise if the incident was a road traffic accident ask if they were wearing a seat belt and note if there is a mark on the skin of the chest caused by one. This is also usually recorded by ambulance crews. Record if the patient has been drinking alcohol and how much and if they smelt of it. A history of headache, nausea or vomiting may be relevant to a head injury or alcohol intoxication.

Before demonstrating a suggested sequence of examining a patient with a possible facial fracture, it is necessary to consider what we are looking for and what symptoms they might have. We will go through the common fractures in terms of their anatomy, symptoms and signs on clinical examination.

Fractures will be considered in the following groups: zygomatic (also called malar) fractures, mandible, dento- alveolar, nasal, and maxillary (also called middle third).

Fractures of the Zygoma (Malar)

The zygomatic fracture is pyramidal shaped and involves the zygoma and adjacent bones. Usually the injury is sustained from a single blow which is usually from a fist. The fracture involves a break at the fronto-zygomatic suture (**A**) which extends through the lateral wall of the orbit and orbital floor (**B**) which is very thin. It then passes though the inferior orbital margin (**C**) to the infra-orbital foramen and then down the zygomatic buttress (**D**) and finally through the zygomatic arch (**E**).

Symptoms

Most patients will have soreness and swelling. Those with severe displacements may have diplopia (double vision). Most will have numbness of the side of the face and difficulty on moving their mandible, particularly laterally.

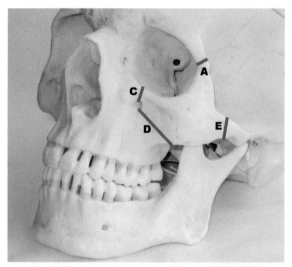

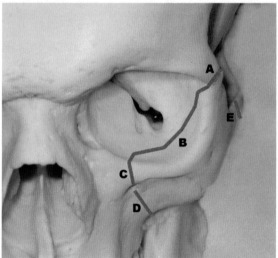

Signs to look for

Initially there may be quite severe swelling and bruising which may be such that assessment may be difficult. Sometimes the eye may be completely closed and it will be necessary to part the eyelids with your fingers to look at it. A crude assessment of vision should be made by asking the patient to count how many fingers you hold up before them. If there is any doubt they should be referred to an ophthalmic surgeon for assessment and opinion. Many patients will have a sub-conjunctival haemorrhage which in itself does not indicate a fracture but it is said that if a posterior limit cannot be seen there is a higher indication of a fracture.

It is quite possible that the patient may have quite severe soft tissue swelling without having a fracture, and in many cases it is best to postpone final

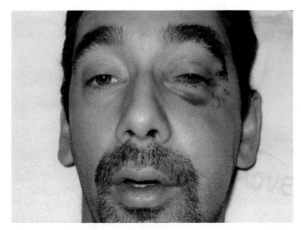

Obvious flattening of left Zygoma

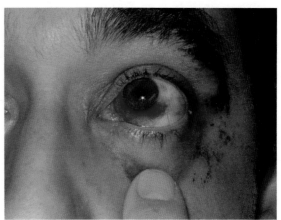

Sub-conjunctival haemorrhage

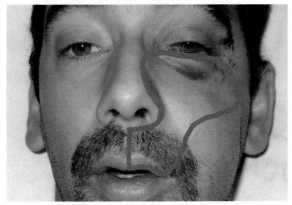

Extent of numbness caused by infra orbital nerve compression

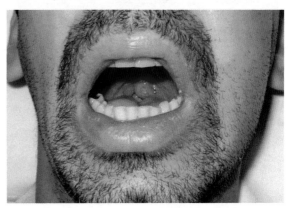

Limitation of opening and lateral jaw movement

assessment for a few days until the swelling has mostly subsided. When making this assessment you should examine for the following features:-

1. Diplopia. You should hold up a finger tip about one metre away and ask the patient to look at it with both eyes and move it throughout the field of vision and ask them to report if they should see double. This may occur if there is disruption of the volume of the orbit in a severe fracture. Diplopia can be measured by an orthoptist in the Ophthalmic Department using a Hess chart.

2. Cosmetic flattening. This may be obvious, but subtle flattening can best be assessed from above by placing a finger on the malar eminence on both sides and comparing.

3. Step deformity on palpation of the margin of the orbital most easily felt at the inferior orbital margin.

4. Numbness in the distribution of the infra orbital nerve i.e. the side of the face and gingivae above the incisors and canine on the affected side. This is due to compression of the nerve in the infra orbital canal.

5. Decreased opening consequent upon the zygomatic arch pressing on the temporalis muscle and coronoid process of the mandible.

Management

Usually fractures of the zygoma are elevated using a 'Gillies lift'. An elevator is placed beneath the zygomatic arch through an incision in the temple. Alternatively a hook can be placed through the cheek. Fixation with a plate increases stability and can be placed at the fronto-zygomatic suture or maxillary buttress fracture. Undisplaced or minimally displaced fractures can be managed conservatively but elevation and fixation improve the rate of recovery of numbness.

Fractures of the Mandible

The mandible can fracture at any point along its length but most frequently this occurs:-

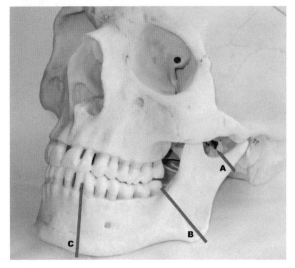

A. At the condyle, usually from a blow to the chin from the opposite side. This is the thinnest and therefore weakest point of the jaw and hence most likely to break.

B. At the angle. Here the bone may be thick but it may be weakened by the presence of an un-erupted or partly erupted third molar.

C. Parasymphyseal

Symptoms

All patients will complain of pain and discomfort; they may feel their teeth are loose; they will have difficulty chewing and may have difficulty biting their teeth together, opening the mouth or moving the jaw sideways.

Signs to look for

Swelling, bruising, cuts, abrasions and tenderness on palpation over mandible and numbness of the lower lip on the affected side. Intra oral examination may reveal loose teeth, missing teeth, bleeding and splits in the gingivae and above all derangement of the occlusion; a haematoma in the floor of the mouth suggests a fracture of the mandibular body. Only a dental surgeon will be able to examine the occlusion and make a judgement about whether it is normal for

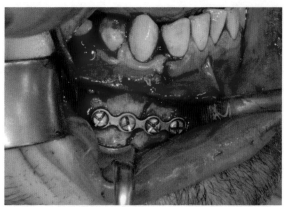

Most mandibular fractures are treated with titanium plates.

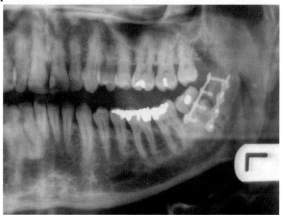

Angle fracture treated with plates - post-op.

that patient; a consideration of the wear facets on the incisal edges and cusps may need to be made.

Management

Most minimally displaced condylar fractures do not have derangement of the occlusion and can be managed conservatively; the patient can be sent home from A&E and reviewed by the Consultant on the clinic. If they are then found to have increasing, rather than improving, pain or occlusal derangement, the jaws can be wired together for two weeks (inter-maxillary fixation) or internally fixed with titanium plates at operation. If the condyles on both sides are fractured the patient is at risk of developing an anterior open bite. The worse of the two fractures is therefore reduced at operation and fixed with a titanium plate then managed as a unilateral case.

Most other fractures of the mandible are admitted to the ward from A&E for reduction and fixation at a

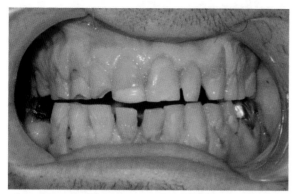

Anterior open bite as a result of bilateral condylar fractures. Obvious only to those with dental training.

convenient time the next day but ideally within 24 hours. Most fractures, other than of the condyles, are compound into the mouth and will therefore be given antibiotics.

Dento-alveolar fractures

Dento-alveolar fractures are a very common sequelae to falls, sporting accidents and interpersonal violence. They will probably correctly be regarded as minor injuries by Accident and Emergency staff. However, long after broken bones have healed and been forgotten about, a patient may continue to suffer the consequences of lost or damaged teeth. Whereas there are good reasons to delay the treatment of more severe facial fractures, dento-alveolar injuries should be managed immediately to ensure the best results. A common cause for complaints concerns patients with dental injuries who are sent away from the Accident and Emergency Department without being referred to OMFS for urgent assessment and management.

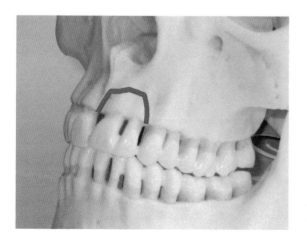

Symptoms

Pain, swelling, bleeding and loose teeth.

Signs to look for

Examine for fractures of the crowns of the teeth, loosening and displacement of the teeth. Look for splits in the attached gingivae. Note which teeth are affected as this may be necessary for legal reports later. Look for associated lacerations of the soft tissues and pieces of tooth substance in lip lacerations. If pieces of tooth are missing and the patient may have lost consciousness a chest X-ray may be necessary to ensure that they have not been inhaled; a low exposure X-ray of overlying soft tissue wounds may demonstrate any tooth substance embedded.

Management

Exposed pulps are dressed with dental cement, and loose teeth are repositioned using local anaesthesia, and a temporary splint made, providing they are not too damaged or the periodontal condition too bad. The patient is then brought back to the outpatient clinic on the next working day and the teeth more definitively splinted, using orthodontic wires attached with acid etch composite. The patient is then discharged to the care of a primary care or restorative dentist for further follow up, assuming there are no other injuries to be attended to. It is usual for periapical X-rays not to be available out of hours but the initial urgent treatment is not usually compromised by this.

Fractures of the Nose

Fractures of the nose are very common and result from interpersonal violence, sporting injuries and falls. Most isolated nasal fractures may be referred directly to the ENT department from the Accident and Emergency Department whereas we tend to get those which accompany other facial fractures, as a matter of convenience. The nasal bones support the nasal cartilages which support the shape of the external nose, and both of these may fracture, as may the cartilage of the nasal septum.

Symptoms

Patients with fractures of the nose may complain of pain, swelling, deformity, bleeding or obstruction of the nasal airway.

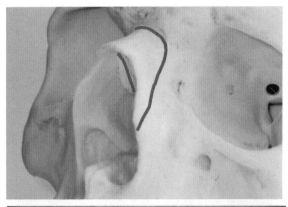

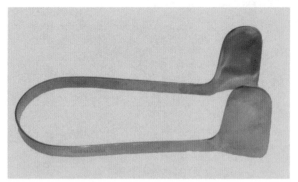

Nasal speculum to examine inside the nose

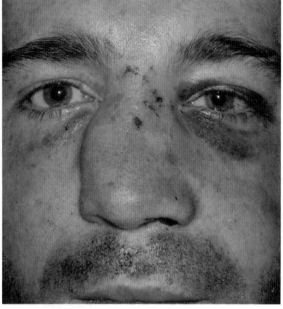

Deviation of dorsum of nose

Signs to look for

The most common complaint will be of nasal deformity and this is best assessed very soon after the injury before soft tissue swelling has developed, or several days later when it has subsided. Occasionally a patient will present who is so annoying that he has received a thumping to the nose on several occasions. In this circumstance a nasal deformity caused by an old injury can be differentiated from a new one by attempting lateral movement of the nose between gloved fingers and thumb; deformity from an old injury will be firm.

The internal nose should be examined with a good light and a nasal speculum. Nasal obstruction may be caused by a blood clot, a deviation of the nasal septum (ask if they had a clear airway before) or a septal haematoma beneath the perichondrium of cartilaginous septum. Although it is unusual, should a haematoma become infected it can cause necrosis of the cartilage which may result in loss of support for the dorsum of the nose, and a saddle nose deformity may result. We suggest that it would be appropriate to ask an ENT surgeon to see the patient in this circumstance.

A special mention for X-rays. These are contraindicated in nasal fractures. X-rays have a low sensitivity and specificity for identifying nasal fractures. Fractures of the cartilage will not be demonstrated at all as may many nasal bone fractures. In addition small vascular markings may appear as fractures to a radiologist and be reported as such when there has been no fracture.

Management

A deviated nose can often be manipulated between fingers and thumb to straighten it without anaesthetic, if done very soon after the injury. A septal haematoma beneath the perichondrium of the cartilaginous septum should be drained using local anaesthetic. Otherwise a deviated nose can be manipulated under general or using local anaesthetic a week later when the swelling has subsided; this will make assessment easier. If the nasal septum remains deviated, causing obstruction to the airway, this is generally managed at a later date by a sub mucous resection of the septum which is a routine operation by an ENT surgeon.

Fractures of the Maxilla

Maxillary, or middle third (of the face) fractures as they are more accurately described, are nowadays infrequent. They can be occasionally caused by very severe interpersonal violence but their heyday, when cars had no seatbelts, crumple zones or airbags, has long passed. We get a slow trickle of these injuries from slow speed accidents involving lorry drivers who are not legally obliged to wear seat belts and who think it is safer to be 'thrown clear' of an accident than strapped into it. In rural areas some very severe injuries can be caused by horse kicks.

Maxillary fractures were classified by a Frenchman called René Le Fort at the beginning of the last century. He smashed 35 faces (the victims were already dead), dissected them and wrote up his findings. He designated mid face fractures as Le Fort 1,2 or 3. The classification does not have a lot of relevance, as in practice the bones are often smashed into small pieces rather than following the lines of his classification. However he captured the imagination of surgeons and his classification has been passed from one generation of surgical textbooks to the next so that most surgeons have heard of it but few will understand it (including many of the authors).

Sometimes when a patient is admitted to an Accident and Emergency Department with a maxillary fracture you may find an orthopaedic, surgical or A&E Specialist Registrar poring over the CT scan or facial X-ray trying to work out whether it is a Le Fort 1, 2 or 3; they expect they might need to know for their forthcoming examinations. You can impress them by telling them that it is a Le Fort 2. This is because most of them are and even if you are wrong they will never find out.

Symptoms

The patients will probably, but not necessarily, have severe facial swelling and bruising, their eyes may be completed closed with oedema, they will have been bleeding from the nose and the mouth and they will have a disturbed occlusion and loose teeth. Many of these injures will have been caused by severe trauma which may have caused other injuries. The patient will probably have a head injury or a neck injury so a cervical collar will have been placed to stabilise the neck and only removed after the neck has been X rayed and examined by an orthopaedic surgeon. The airway may be at risk so the patient may have been intubated. Generally speaking the facial injuries themselves will not be life threatening so other injuries will take priority.

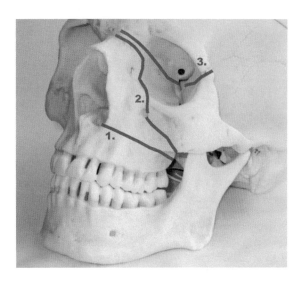

Le Fort Classification: 1. Low level, separates the dento-alveolar segment from the rest of the maxilla, is very unusual as it requires a severe force in a very concentrated area of the lower part of maxilla above the teeth. 2. The most common. It is a pyramidal fracture across nasal bones, through orbits and across buttress of the zygoma. 3. Separation of whole of face from cranial base, a very severe injury; many with this may not survive the head injury. The pattern may be different on each side, there may be fractures at several levels on the same side, and the bones may be comminuted into small pieces.

Signs to look for

Examination may be difficult if the patient is intubated and wearing a cervical collar. If not intubated examine the dentition and occlusion, examine for numbness and look at the eyes to check vision is OK. The diagnosis of maxillary fracture is easily made by holding the anterior maxilla with a gloved hand and attempting a differential movement of the maxilla while holding the bridge of the nose between the finger and thumb of the other hand.**Management**

Definitive surgery for a maxillary fracture may be delayed for a couple of weeks while the swelling subsides and other injuries are dealt with, in particular orthopaedic injuries and recovery from head injury.

Very occasionally, bleeding from the maxilla will be difficult to control, in which case you will need to call someone senior. Patients with head injuries will probably need a CT scan and the most useful thing you can do is ask them to include the face in the initial scan. Coronal views showing the orbital floor and volume will be most useful.

Although definitive surgery may be delayed it may be necessary to take them to theatre that day to do a tracheotomy to secure the airway, in which case loose teeth can be removed, severely displaced fractures can be temporarily approximated with wires, and lacerations sutured.

Definitive surgery may vary from as little as a couple of plates placed within the mouth for a patient with an intact dental arch and little displacement of the occlusion, to major surgery involving open reduction of the fractures from both intra and extra oral approaches, and taking most of a day.

Now that we have very briefly described the main types of facial fractures that you will come across you should have a rough idea what you are looking for. We will now go through a sequence of the steps you should go through when you see a patient with facial trauma.

Examination of the face

1. Examine soft tissues

Draw a rough diagram of lacerations, abrasions and other skin marks and include measurements.

2. Examine the eyes

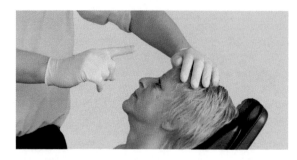

Look for sub-conjunctival haemorrhage (redness below the conjunctiva), and level of the pupil compared with the opposite side. Steady the patient's head and ask them to follow your finger, held one metre away, through all movements to check ocular movements (particularly upwards) and ask if they have any double vision.

Before examining the face

Take a history

 Record the time you saw them

Can they remember the incident?
How did the injury occur?
Time of injury
Anyone else hurt?
Wearing seat belt?
Alcohol involved?
Past medical history
Social history

Direct questions

 Headache

Any loss of consciousness?
Nausea or vomiting?
Vision OK? Diplopia
Numbness of face
Police involvement

Also examine & record

 Injuries elsewhere

Glasgow coma scale
(in practice this will already have been done by casualty doctor before you were called.)

A malar fracture may cause sub-conjunctival bleeding; a severe fracture may cause a lowering of the orbital floor and hence the globe of the eye. A large change in orbital volume in such an injury can lead to diplopia and may entrap orbital contents (particularly inferior rectus muscle) in the fractured floor, causing limitation of upward gaze.

3. Palpate the orbital margins

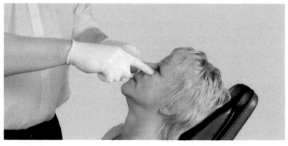

Palpate the orbital rims for evidence of a step deformity which would be felt if there were a fracture of the Zygoma or much less commonly a Le Fort 2 of the maxilla.

4. Look for flattening of the Zygoma

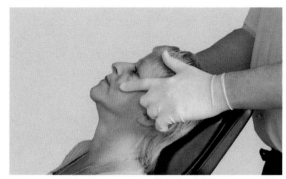

This is best achieved by standing behind the patient and looking and palpating the prominence of the cheek and comparing the two sides. Flattening is best assessed either very soon after the injury, before swelling has started, or several days later when it has started to subside.

5. Check nose

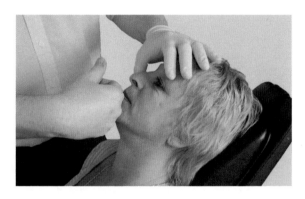

Is the nose deviated and if so does this predate the injury or is it new? Check the nasal airway by obstructing each nostril in turn and feeling for the breath with your finger.

6. Examine inside the nose

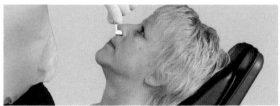

Use a nasal speculum to look for a septal swelling which may be a haematoma needing draining. Don't bother if there is no obvious nasal injury.

7. Examine for numbness

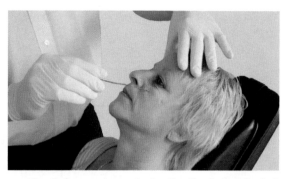

Check for numbness in the distribution of the infra orbital nerve on the face which usually accompanies a malar or maxillary fracture. Remember not to miss the gingivae above the incisor and canine teeth which will be involved. The mental nerve may have been injured in fractures of the mandible.

8. Is the maxilla firm ?

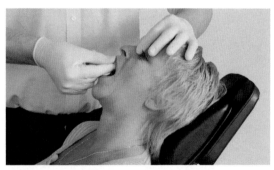

Wearing gloves, hold the nasal bridge and anterior maxillary alveolus firmly and try to elicit a differential movement

9. Examine the mouth

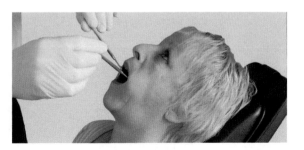

Look for loose and broken teeth, derangement of the occlusion, tears in the soft tissues and particularly of the gingivae. Using gloved hands, try to elicit movement across any part of the mandible you suspect may be fractured but are not sure. Check for mouth opening and lateral movement. Feel for tenderness of the temporomandibular joint.

Glasgow Coma Scale

The GCS is frequently used to describe the state of a head injury. You will see it noted in the Accident and Emergency records of most patients attending after severe trauma. A score of 15 is normal.

Score the following and add:

Eye Response. (Possible total 4)

1. No eye opening
2. Eye opening to pain
3. Eye opening to verbal command
4. Eyes open spontaneously

Verbal Response (Possible total 5)

1. No verbal response
2. Incomprehensible sounds
3. Inappropriate words
4. ? Confused
5. ? Orientated

Motor Response (Possible total 6)

1. No motor response
2. Extension to pain
3. Flexion to pain.
4. Withdrawal from pain
5. Localising pain
6. Obeys Commands

Score of 15: normal
13+: mild brain injury
9 - 12: moderate injury
8 or less: severe brain injury

An example of what to write.

29.6.13   00.15 Hr.
Robert Andrews 20♂
– alleged assault at approx 10.00 pm.
2 blows to left side of face
– not been drinking can remember incident
LOC°   nausea°   vomiting°
only facial injury
o/e alert & orientated GCS=15
° SC haemorrhage, normal eye movement
° diplopia   ° malar flattening
Nasal airway patient
maxilla firm
° facial numbness
   left lip swollen, 2 cm laceration through skin & vermillion of lip – not throu to mouth

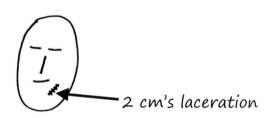

2 cm's laceration

<u>IOE</u>

Mobility between 12

 1 # enamel just into dentine

Premature occlusion L buccal

segment

° floor mouth haematoma

<u>OPG</u>

Confirms # R parasymphysis

Between 1 & 2

<u>Plan</u>

Inform specialist registrar on call

1.   Suture laceration LA

1.   Admit to ward

1.   IV fluid

1.   Nil by mouth for theatre

am

<u>Treat</u>

LA lidocaine/adrenaline

1 X 2.0 mls cartridge

2 cm laceration closed with deep

3/0 Vicryl & 5/0 ethylon to skin

R Undergreen.

ROB UNDERGREEN

OMFS FT2

22. Imaging for Facial Fractures

The majority of patients with fractures of the facial skeleton will have the fracture diagnosed from the history and symptoms confirmed by clinical examination. In practically all cases an X-ray examination will be made to confirm the diagnosis and to aid in the planning of surgery. For fractures of the mandible the orthopantomograph (OPG) will combine the most radiological information with best radiological hygiene. In most cases the OPG alone will suffice but some fractures of the angle or condyle will not be visualized and a posterior-anterior (PA) image will be used as well. Although most cases will be obvious from clinical examination many surgeons will feel more comfortable having two images at right angles.

You will already be aware that the OPG is a tomogram, the principle of which is that the X-ray source and sensor rotate around the subject so that radiopaque structures (cervical spine in this case) not of interest are outside the focal trough. This decreases interference with the image of the area being examined. The main limitation of the OPG for trauma patients is that the patient must be able to stand or sit in the machine, so it may not be suitable for those with severe or multiple injuries, especially if they are wearing a cervical collar because of a possible neck injury. In these cases a CT scan will be used, the patient will almost certainly be having a CT for their other injuries anyway. If you arrive on the scene early ask them to extend the CT to include the face, if this has not already been done.

For the PA view of the mandible the X-ray sensor or film plate is placed in front of the face and the rays pass from behind the patient forward at 90° to the sensor.

The other common facial fracture is of the malar (zygoma). CT scans are usually used by most surgeons for all mid-face fractures but you may well find that many feel comfortable managing simple malar fractures with just a plain X-ray. The image used will be the 15° occipito-mental (OM). Here the principle is that X-rays will pass through the occiput to the sensor which is at 15° to the perpendicular of the film. The patient is positioned with his chin and nose touching the sensor. This should produce a clear image of the bony margins of the mid face. The patient must be able to stand, sit or lie face down. An image made with the patient lying on his back and the film behind the head

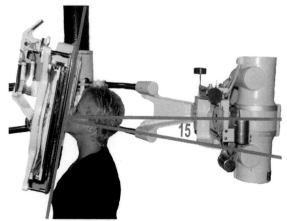

Making 15° OM image

will give an indistinct view of the mid face.

In most cases where you are asked to see a patient with facial trauma images will have already have been obtained. If not, an OPG and 15° OM are all you need to request. It will be unusual for someone at a junior level to have the authority to order CT scans but your chief may well want them. Remember it is always good practice to get into the habit of examining the patient and making a clinical diagnosis before looking at images.

Computerized Tomography (CT) is an X-ray image made using the tomography principle. The X-ray source and sensors are located in a ring which spirals around the patient as they move through on a platform. In older scanners the image is acquired in an axial plain, and coronal and sagittal scans are reconstructed by the computer. With modern scans a 3D data set is used and the image can be viewed in three dimensions giving the surgeon a more realistic image in what will be encountered at operation. This is of particular value in fractures around the orbit.

Do not miss the opportunity to see CT scans being made; the best way to see the images is on the video screen in the scanner centre with the radiologist or the radiographer demonstrating to you. The traditional technique of printing images onto film is now obsolete as digital imaging systems are built into hospitals using video screens to view images.

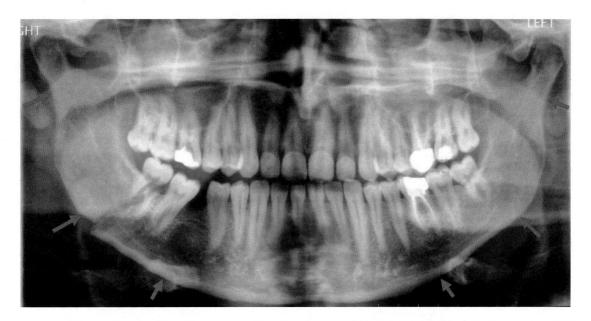

Always check the name of the patient on the film, the date and orientation. Examine all the margins of the mandible sequentially, the most common sites of fracture being the condylar neck, angle and parasymphysis. Check that your diagnosis fits with the clinical findings. The fracture here is obvious at the right angle involving the second molar tooth. The fracture is often seen as a double lucency which represents the break through the buccal and lingual cortex of the mandible, and not two separate fractures.

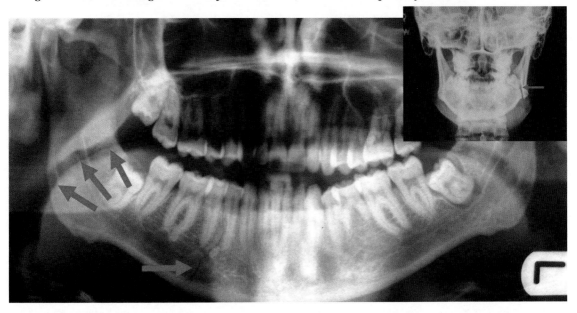

OPG Potential Problems: *To the untutored observer who has not properly examined the patient the pharyngeal air shadow can sometimes be suspected as a fracture. This is marked at the right angle, however you can see that it extends beyond the mandible. The fracture marked at the right body is clear but can you see a fracture at the left angle? No, neither can we. However, a PA view (X rays passing from posterior to anterior) clearly shows the fracture. Sometimes an angle fracture will not show clearly. However, this will be suspected from clinical examination and the taking of a PA film as a routine is not justified. The OPG does not image the symphysis well because of the superimposition of the cervical spine. This can be imaged with an intra-oral occlusal film.*

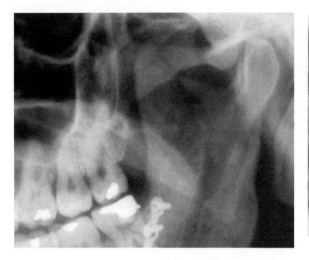

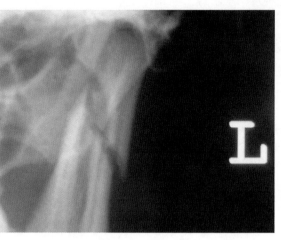

Detail from an OPG shows the condylar fracture but ...

... it is more clearly seen on the detail from the PA film.

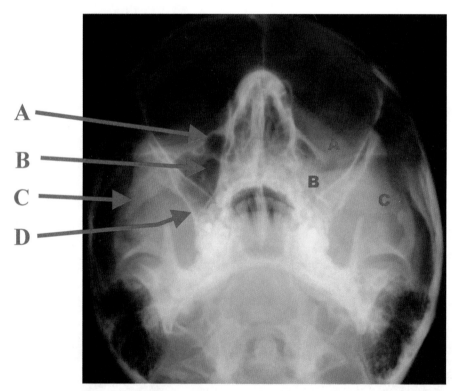

15° Occipital-mental of patient with fracture of left malar. Compare the injured with the uninjured side, looking at: A. The rim of the orbit for loss of continuity. B. The maxillary antrum for a fluid level or opacity caused by blood. . C. The zygomatic arch D. The lateral maxillary wall for loss of continuity. You can see that on the left side there is severe disruption of the orbital rim, loss of opacity of the antrum, a break in the zygomatic arch, and it is difficult to make out the lateral antral wall clearly. A widening of the fronto-zygomatic suture is also frequently seen in zygomatic fractures. However, the suture can often be quite prominent anyway if the x-rays are angled with the film so as to accentuate it.

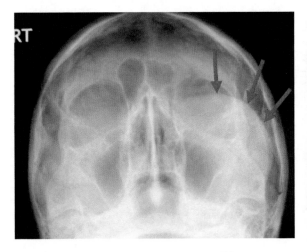

15° OM potential problems. The maxillary antrum may appear opaque from severe facial swelling or haematoma in the soft tissues. Look for soft tissue shadow as marked above.

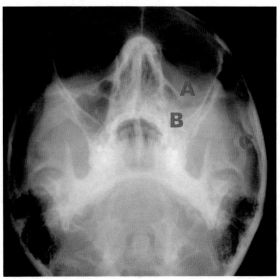

15° OM. A. Buckled orbital rim B. Opaque maxillary antrum due to blood and displaced bone from lateral antral wall C. Fracture of zygomatic arch

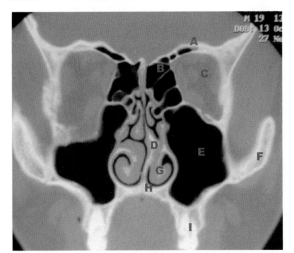

Coronal CT of mid face. A. Cranial base B. Ethmoidal air cells C. Orbit (behind the globe of the eye), the medial, lateral, superior and inferior rectus muscles and the optic nerve may be seen as slight opacities D. Nasal septum (deviated) E. Maxillary antrum F. Prominence of Zygoma G. Inferior concha H. Bony palate I. Molar tooth

The scan shows an isolated fracture of the right orbital floor (orbital blow out) with part of the orbital contents bulging into the maxillary antrum.

Let us compare the quality and clarity of the 15° occipito-mental plain x-ray 3-D images, axial CT slice and 3-D CT image of a patient who has suffered a fractured malar (zygoma).

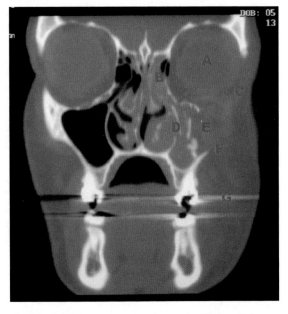

Coronal CT scan same patient. A. Globe of the eye in the same position as uninjured side B. Ethmoids filled with opaque blood, inferior orbital wall fractured C. Prominence of Zygoma missing from same plane as uninjured side D. Blood in the nose and lateral nasal wall fractured E. Bone and blood in the antrum F Lateral antral wall missing G. Artefacts from amalgam fillings

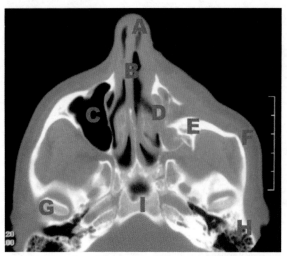

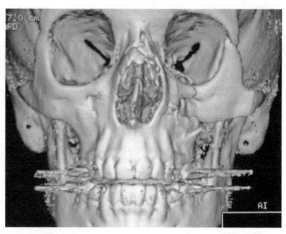

Axial CT scan of the same patient. A. External nose B. Nasal septum C. Maxillary antrum on uninjured side D. Position of antrum on injured side showing opaque blood and bone fragments within E. Prominence of Zygoma displaced inwards F. Zygomatic arch G. Condyles of mandible H. Mastoid air cells I. Cervical spine

The computer can be used to adjust the view of the 3-D image. Note the artifacts caused by amalgam fillings.

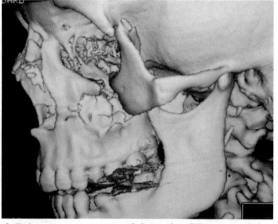

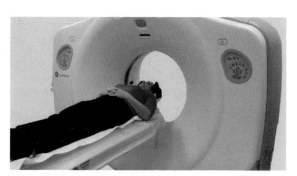

Patient in CT scanner

3-D image reconstructed from the CT scans of the same patient with fracture of the right malar.

23. <u>Admitting a Patient with a Facial Fracture</u>

Most patients who present to you from the A&E Department with facial fractures will require hospital admission, but not quite all.

Some surgeons may prefer to operate upon fractures of the malar complex (zygoma) at a later stage when the swelling has gone down and so the patient will not need to be in hospital for a few days. As long as they have been cleared from having any head injury and their eyes are uninjured they can be discharged home with an appointment to be reviewed in the outpatient clinic by the Consultant at a convenient time. In busy units with a high trauma load there may be regular dedicated trauma clinics for this purpose. The same applies to unilateral mandibular condyle, orbital blow out and isolated nasal fractures which will not necessarily need immediate hospitalization.

It will also be necessary for you to make arrangements for patients to be reviewed who have sustained facial trauma but not any obvious fracture or soft tissue injury. You may soon become proficient at examining patients and interpreting facial x-ray and CT images but the Consultant will be better so it is wise that he or she has the opportunity to check to make sure you have not missed something.

Nearly all mandibular fractures will need hospital admission. The standard management for mandibular fractures is open reduction and fixation with titanium plates which should preferably be done within 24 hours of injury. Once you have made the diagnosis you should inform your superior so that they can arrange to see the patient at an appropriate time. A ward bed should be found (which should not be your job) and the patient admitted. Accurate notes should be made as described in the previous chapters and the patient and any accompanying friends or relatives made aware of what the plan is.

Having made an arrangement with your superior of when and where surgery is to take place the operating theatre and anaesthetist should be informed of the presence of the patient. The anaesthetist will want to know of the patient's general health and if they can open their mouth easily as this will have a bearing on the anaesthetic (see anaesthetic chapter).

All mandibular fractures (apart from condylar) are compound into the mouth so it is normal practice for the patients to be prescribed antibiotics to reduce the risk of infection which is heightened by the fact that a foreign body (titanium plate) is going to be placed into the fracture. The patient will need to be 'nil by mouth' because they will be having a general anaesthetic and so will need an IV infusion to give them fluids and the antibiotics will be given IV as well, usually Co-Amoxiclav. 2½ litres of fluid should be prescribed on a fluid chart to run over 24 hours and if the patient has been drinking alcohol they will already be a little dehydrated so the quantity should be increased (see fluids section of prescribing chapter).

All patients with mid face maxillary fractures will need hospital admission. These fractures require a substantial force to produce so you should assume the patient has some form of head injury associated with it and that there might be a neck injury so the neck should be imaged and cleared by an orthopaedic surgeon or trauma team before the neck is moved substantially without the patient wearing a neck collar to protect it.

Very few facial injuries are life threatening so immediate surgery is required in proportionally few cases. However, in severe injuries there may be significant bleeding, loose teeth or associated soft tissue injuries which may compromise the airway. In these cases the first contact with the patient may be in the resuscitation room in A&E where there will be an anaesthetist who has already sedated and intubated the patient. In this scenario they will want a tracheostomy to ensure no airway obstruction. In this case the surgeon will operate straight away to do the tracheostomy, remove severely damaged or loose teeth and arrest haemorrhage. This raises an interesting consent issue. The patient cannot give consent themselves as they are not conscious. The surgeon should concur with a colleague to agree that this is necessary to avoid risk of loss of life. But what about the fracture of the mandible which could easily wait a day or two? It seems a nonsense to leave it and wake the patient up to get their consent to do the operation which they will need anyway when they are already in the operating theatre. The law is an ass.

<table>
<tr><td>

<u>*Key Points*</u>

• No admission required for zygomatic, unilateral mandibular condylar or isolated nasal fractures with no head or eye injury

• Check facial imaging with your 2nd on call or supervisor to ensure no undiagnosed fractures

• All other mandibular fractures require hospital admission – contact your superior and inform bed manager

</td><td>

• All mandibular fractures (except isolated condylar) are compound into the mouth – prescribe antibiotics, 'nil by mouth', IV infusion and plan for surgery

• All maxillary (midface) fractures require hospital admission – high impact force - clear neck injury with trauma or orthopaedic team

• Severe facial injuries can compromise airway – significant bleeding and soft tissue injuries, loose teeth or foreign bodies – immediate surgery

</td></tr>
</table>

24. <u>Admitting a Patient with a Dental Abscess</u>

Many patients attend A&E departments with dental pain. It is not the duty of A&E or OMFS to relieve the primary care dental services of the pleasure or responsibility of relieving pain. However among these patients will be a number who have an abscess with pus formation which could cause systemic illness or even loss of life eventually should it progress unchecked.

Patients with apical periodontitis or small abscesses can be advised to seek urgent care from a primary dentist the next day or if deteriorating from your own out-patient clinic the next day.

A few patients with advanced abscesses will need hospital admission for removal of the causative tooth and drainage of pus. Nearly all of these patients will have been seen in a primary care facility and been prescribed antibiotics. Sometimes they may have been seen by a medical practitioner who is unable to do anything else to help but more usually they have seen a dentist who simply cannot be bothered to remove or drain the tooth properly. Often we see patients who have re-presented to the dentist with a worsening abscess unresponsive to antibiotics, only to leave with a different antibiotic or the dose doubled. We have seen numerous cases over the years where the dentist has told a patient that they cannot do anything until the swelling has resolved. In dental schools students are encouraged to use antibiotics inappropriately, usually taught by dentists who have not worked in OMFS departments and seen the consequence of inappropriate antibiotic prescription. In general dental practice it is possible to get away with antibiotic use in some cases which encourages over prescription; it makes financial

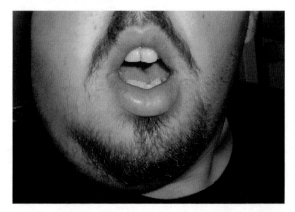

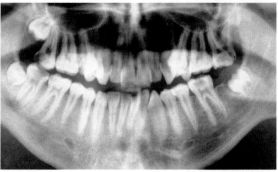

Patient with pain at LR7 presented to dentist who could'nt be bothered to remove the tooth and instead prescribed two antibiotics over two weeks. Now he has trismus and extra-oral swelling and needs admission for removal of the tooth and extra-oral drainage. Such negligence is commonplace.

sense to a practitioner to fob patients off with a quick script rather than interrupt the smooth process of accumulating cash or 'units of dental activity' by taking time to treat an urgent case properly.

A patient should be admitted to hospital if they have any of the following symptoms: firm swelling (rather than just soft oedematous), limitation of mouth opening, difficulty in swallowing, swelling extending down the neck, facial swelling extending up to the eye.

Full notes should be made which should include a dental assessment and OPG image requested. It is usual, but not essential, for a full blood count which will probably show an increased white cell count depending upon the systemic upset caused by the abscess. A sample for biochemistry urea and electrolytes should be taken; this should include a glucose estimation as there is a possibility that some degree of compromised immunity may be the result of undiagnosed diabetes. The patient's temperature should be taken and this should be repeated every six hours. Pyrexia is to be expected and indicates systemic upset; where there is un-drained pus present the pattern seen on the temperature chart will be 'swinging' with the temperature going up and down. Once the pus is drained the temperature should dip and stay down.

Once on the ward the patient should have an IV drip; if they are pyrexial they will have an increased insensible loss of fluid so will need more than the standard 2½ litres over 24 hours and they may be somewhat dehydrated if they have not been eating and drinking normally because of pain or swelling.

For a patient who is unwell enough to need hospital admission an antibiotic is appropriate but is not the definitive treatment. A broad spectrum antibiotic active against the gram negative organisms normally present should be given intravenously. This would normally be co-amoxiclav or metronidazole. The antibiotic has the effect of limiting the spread of pus through the soft tissues so that it becomes localised and therefore easier to drain surgically. The patient will also need analgesia.

In most cases 24 hours of IV antibiotics will be sufficient to localise the swelling and the causative tooth should be removed and pus drained. If the patient can open their mouth sufficiently the tooth can be removed and pus drained with local anaesthetic. However most cases will need to be done in the operating theatre; the anaesthetist will need to know about limited mouth opening so that someone skilled in dealing with this can be involved (see anaesthetic chapter).

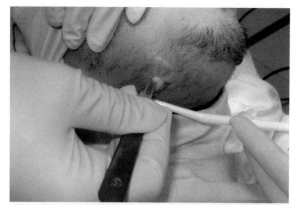
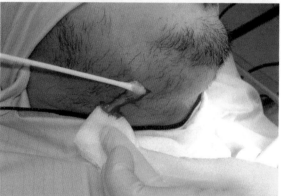
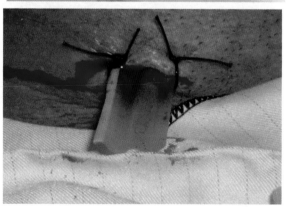

After incision and drainage a swab is usually taken for microbiology culture and sensitivity and a drain sewed in to facilitate drainage of pus.

In theatre the tooth should be removed and pus drained. It is normal practice for a swab of the pus to be sent to the laboratory for culture and antibiotic sensitivity but we have found this rarely has any impact on the patient's management as once the pus is drained they improve and usually don't require antibiotics. However it is normal practice to change the antibiotics to oral administration at this stage rather than stop them altogether and to stop them completely when the patient goes home in a day or two. If an extra-oral incision has been made to drain the pus we normally sew in a plastic drain to facilitate drainage and prevent the skin from healing over the pus; this is normally secured to the skin with one or two silk sutures.

If the patient has a very neglected mouth it may be appropriate to remove all teeth that are past restoration under the same anaesthetic. However it may not be in the patient's best interest to cause the increased bleeding this will involve if their trismus is severe, and the anaesthetist and operating theatre staff may not be happy for you to spend over an hour doing a difficult full or part dental clearance if there are other cases waiting for time on an 'emergency' operating list.

Once the patient is able to eat and drink enough to get sufficient calories and fluid and they are able to care for themselves they may be discharged home. They do not need to stay in hospital until all the pus has drained out; they can be given dressings to take home to mop up draining pus, and the district nurses can be called upon to help with this. It is usual to remove drains before the patient is discharged but not essential; they can return to the out-patient clinic for this. Remember early discharge from hospital is desirable for other patients as the presence of pus on the ward is an infection risk to everybody.

A review of the patient in the clinic is needed after treatment of an extensive abscess in order to access extra-oral wound healing and for the rare occasions of recurrent infection.

Key Points

• Dental pain – provide sympathy and ibuprofen

• Patients with advanced abscesses – hospital admission – removal of causative tooth and drainage of pus – intra-oral and/or extra-oral

• Adverse signs requiring hospital admission – firm facial swelling, trismus, difficulty in swallowing, swelling extending to neck or eye

• Full history and examination, OPG image, check patient's temperature, blood tests including glucose, intravenous drip, antibiotics, anaesthetic assessment, drainage in operating theatre

• Extra oral drainage requires securing a plastic drain to the skin with sutures

• Change IV to oral antibiotics after successful drainage of pus

• It is optional to remove all other unrestorable teeth

• Remove drain before discharging patient even though some wounds may continue to discharge

25. <u>You Should Know About Retrobulbar Haemorrhage</u>

An unusual but significant complication of major trauma is a haemorrhage behind the globe of the eye causing compression on the optic nerve. This may occur after a major traumatic injury or sometimes as a result of a more minor impact directly to the eye. You should be aware of this injury as its recognition and prompt management are essential; otherwise permanent blindness to the affected eye may result.

The signs are proptosis (protrusion of the globe), blindness of the eye, pain and opthalmoplegia (inability to move the eye). The patient should be treated with high dose steroids and immediate lateral canthotomy and inferior cantholysis to relieve the pressure in the orbit.

Should you see these signs you should call your Specialist Registrar or Consultant and advise them of your concern.

When this patient was brought into A&E no one suspected a retrobulbar haemorrhage or had even examined his eyesight; the main concern was his airway and head injury. The haemorrhage was diagnosed when he was in the CT scanner and subsequent clinical examination confirmed he was blind in the left eye.

The orbit was decompressed by lateral canthotomy in Accident and Emergency under local anaesthetic and he was given high dose steroids . This was carried out 2½ hours after the injury. He could detect light by the following morning and sight was returned within two days. Much further delay would have meant permanent blindness in that eye.

Early examination and suspicion in peri-orbital trauma can save sight. It is unusual however.

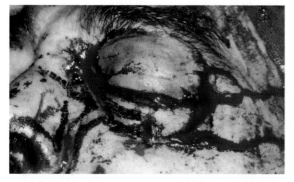

Patient with proptosis, pain opthalmoplegia. There is no sight in the eye.

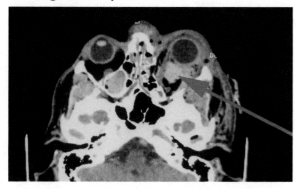

A CT scan shows the collection of blood behind the globe of the eye.

26. <u>Medical Emergencies</u>

The management of medical emergencies and resuscitation is considered very important by the General Dental Council (GDC) and all NHS hospital trusts. You will almost certainly be required to undertake continuing training in these subjects during your time in the hospital for which you are likely to be given a written certificate to prove that you have received it. Make sure that you keep this as it will be necessary for proving that you have undertaken Continuing Professional Development to the GDC; it will also be necessary for your appraisals and in the future revalidation with the GDC.

A medical emergency is a sudden or unexpected event which is potentially life threatening.

You are most likely to have to deal with a medical emergency in the outpatient clinic, possibly when you are carrying out minor surgery using local anaesthetic. Although the chance of this happening is low, it is still higher than when working in dental practice because many patients will be referred to the hospital for minor oral surgery as they have co-existing medical problems. The fact that the situations to be described are either unusual or rare makes it all the more important that you should be up to date with the procedures necessary to recognise and deal with them. You should also know how adverse events might be minimized.

You should be familiar with the recommendations of the Resuscitation Council who provide a document on their web site on the practice and training for cardiopulmonary resuscitation in primary dental care. These guidelines are reviewed regularly and updated according to available evidence; they should be your bible for resuscitation throughout your career and should be memorized for postgraduate examinations as well as for practice. However these recommendations are for a dental surgery and assume no familiarity with gaining intra-venous access. In the hospital IV access will be second nature and there should be a 'medical emergency team' who can be called in all cases where a patient is in danger. They have replaced the concept of the 'cardiac arrest' team who were called when a patient arrested. The medical emergency team are there to act before the patient is in extremis and prevent cardiac arrest as well as managing it wherever possible.

All the equipment needed for dealing with these emergencies should be in the resuscitation trolley, there should be one available in each clinical area including the wards and outpatient departments. This will include drugs, airways and IV access equipment.

Vaso-vagal syncope

In itself vaso-vagal syncope is unlikely to be life threatening but it has to be considered here because it is the most common cause of loss of consciousness in the surgery. It is therefore the first consideration when a patient undergoing a procedure loses consciousness. The diagnosis is easy because it is usually preceded by characteristic prodromal symptoms of light-headedness, feeling hot, sweating and restlessness, often involving rubbing of the face. Recovery is rapid once the patient is tipped back in the chair so that their legs are higher than their head; this can be accelerated by lifting their legs up. In practice we find that loss of consciousness is usually prevented by tipping the patient in response to the prodromal signs.

If the patient actually loses consciousness because the prodromal signs have been missed they may start convulsing; this quickly ceases when consciousness recovers and should not be considered as an epileptic fit.

The process occurs as a result of vagus activity causing a slowing of the heart accompanied by vasodilation producing a decrease in cerebral blood flow. In the oral surgery setting this is most likely to occur when minor oral surgery is performed on a patient who has not eaten for some time and is very apprehensive about the surgery. The reaction is likely

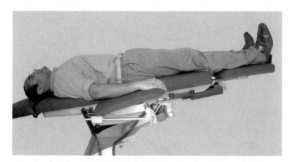

Your first action should be to tip the chair or operating table down so that the patient's legs are raised.

to be triggered by pain, prolonged operating time and the negative emotion of loss of confidence in the surgeon's ability to achieve adequate analgesia. An apprehensive patient may react to the tactile pressure of exodontia as if in pain, even if optimal anaesthesia has been obtained; this may be exacerbated by repeatedly poking the area and asking if they can feel it. An inexperienced or bad nurse assistant can almost talk a patient into passing out by repeatedly asking after their welfare during the operation.

Recovery can be helped by providing oxygen through a face mask. Once consciousness is regained treatment can then be finished with the patient in a slightly reclined or horizontal position.

Other relatively benign causes of loss of consciousness are postural hypotension and hyperventilation. Postural hypotension usually occurs as a result of standing up rapidly, usually pre-disposed to by anti-hypertensive medication. Hyperventilation resulting from anxiety can cause light headedness but rarely loss of consciousness.

Anaphylaxis

Anaphylaxis is a severe allergic reaction resulting in IgE mediated de-granulation of mast cells with the release of histamine. The histamine causes vasodilatation of arterioles and bronchospasm leading to decrease in blood pressure and respiratory distress. The decrease in blood pressure may proceed to collapse and cardiac arrest. The bronchospasm may proceed to respiratory arrest and be followed by cardiac arrest.

Anaphylaxis may result from allergy to a medication or its additives. It may result from systemic or topical administration or even to latex gloves.

The patient may (or may not) have a flushed

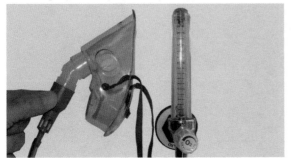

Oxygen should be available on the wall of all the surgeries you use.

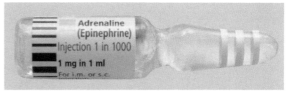

Adrenaline. 1:1000 for anaphylaxis

appearance, urticaria, angioedema, vomiting, wheezing, stridor, hoarse voice and loss of consciousness. The reaction may vary from mild producing little more than a flushed appearance, to cardiopulmonary arrest and death.

In severe cases the patient should be reclined, given oxygen at 15 L/min. and 0.5 mls. of 1:1000 adrenaline intramuscularly into the antero-lateral thigh. The medical emergency team should be called. The adrenaline may be repeated after five minutes if blood pressure or adequate respiration are not maintained. An intravenous line should be put in quickly, and Hartmann's solution or 0.9% saline given to restore blood pressure. Antihistamines and steroids may be given initially in milder cases or after resuscitation in more severe cases. Immediate resuscitation according to the ABCDE approach (see next chapter) will be needed if there is loss of consciousness or breathing stops.

Asthma and COPD

You will have to see a large number of patients who suffer from asthma or Chronic Obstructive Pulmonary Disease (COPD). Most patients will be very knowledgeable about the pattern and severity of their disease. In the unlikely circumstance that a patient suffers an acute exacerbation of their asthma

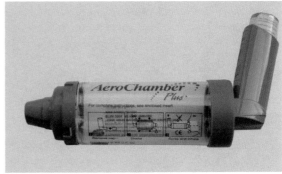

Salbutamol inhaler attached to a spacer which improves the efficiency of drug delivery to the airways.

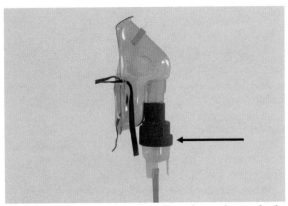

Salbutamol, placed in a nebuliser (arrow) attached to a standard face mask and air supply, is the most efficient way to dilate the airways in severe asthma.

in the clinic or during minor surgery they will usually respond to salbutamol delivered through their own inhaler. If they are very short of breath they may not be able to inhale an adequate dose from an inhaler alone, in which case it may be necessary to use a spacer to deliver the salbutamol.

If the asthma is severe as indicated by the patient's inability to speak a sentence in one breath or they have a respiratory rate increased to 25 per minute or more, or a tachycardia of more than 110 per minute, they will need salbutamol and oxygen through a nebuliser. By this stage you should have called the medical emergency team.

You will occasionally see patients with COPD which is so severe that they use regular home nebulisers or oxygen. In these circumstances their minor surgery or dental extractions are best done under local anaesthetic in the operating theatre, under the supervision of an anaesthetist with oxygen administered with nasal cannulae, heart monitoring, an IV line and possibly some light sedation.

Epilepsy

You would normally be aware of a patient with epilepsy from taking their previous medical history. Most are very well controlled but you should still be aware of what to do if a patient should have a grand-mal seizure. This should be fairly easy to recognise. Before becoming unconscious the patient may have a brief 'aura' which is followed by rigidity and possibly cyanosis, after which there will be jerking movements of the limbs and possible urinary incontinence. The attack may last for a few minutes

and be followed by floppiness. Eventually they become conscious again but possibly confused.

The patient should be given oxygen at 15 L/min. while fitting, and attempts should be made to avoid them injuring themselves. However they should not be physically restrained and nothing should be put into their mouth, not even an oral airway. If fitting continues for longer than five minutes buccal midazolam should be administered and IV access established. If the patient needs such medication to control the fit they will need hospital admission and a review by the medical team. If the fitting continues the medical emergency team should be called, they would normally give IV lorazepam as the next line in management. Occasionally a fit may be triggered by hypoglycaemia so the blood sugar should be checked and if below 3 mmols./ L glucose or glucagon should be given as described below.

Should a patient remain unresponsive after the fit and has no sign of breathing or pulse, Cardio Pulmonary Resuscitation should be started according to the ABCDE principle (described in next chapter).

Hypoglycaemia

Diabetic patients will normally be able to recognise the symptoms of hypoglycaemia. They will feel a general uneasiness and malaise with fatigue and nervousness. This can normally be reversed quickly by taking a drink containing glucose; milk with three teaspoons of sugar added will be very suitable or a sweet (not low calorie) drink or snack. If the symptoms are not recognised it may progress to trembling, headache, tachycardia, aggression, confusion, convulsions and coma. A blood glucose estimation will confirm a level of below 3 mmols. per litre. However, as soon as these signs are seen in a diabetic patient, they should be given a glucose drink if they can swallow.

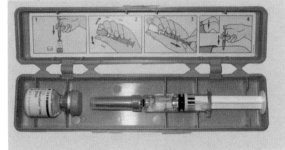

Glucagon pre-loaded in syringe for emergency injection

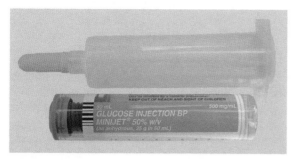

Glucose injection

If the patient should become unconscious they should be given either glucagon, 1 mg. intramuscularly, or 50 mls. of intravenous glucose through a large bore needle. Glucagon is preferable as the glucose solution is highly irritant if any of it is inadvertently injected outside of the vein. This will be needed very rarely as most cases will respond to a glucose drink and the emergency team will not be needed.

Acute Coronary Syndromes

Many patients will be referred into hospital for routine dental extraction simply because they have a history of ischaemic heart disease. A patient with angina will probably carry their own glyceryl trinitrate (GTN) sublingual spray and should they feel any chest pain may well be able to use it to get relief. If this is not unusual for them they can continue with their treatment. In any case where the pain is prolonged the patient should be given oxygen through a face mask and transferred to the Accident and Emergency department or Medical Admissions Unit for an ECG and assessment by a physician.

Patients who have stable angina or a history of a previous myocardial infarct may be treated under local anaesthetic quite satisfactorily in the outpatient facility. However, where there is unstable angina, a history of a very recent infarction or severe heart failure, treatment should be carried out in the operating theatre using local anaesthetic with an anaesthetist supervising their cardiac status with an ECG and giving oxygen with a nasal cannula. Remember that a diabetic or someone elderly may experience only limited pain with a myocardial infarction, or even none at all; your threshold for referral for a medical opinion must be low. In every case of chest pain you should keep an eye on their pulse and respiratory rate. A pulse rate over 100 should be regarded with suspicion, and a respiratory rate of over 15 per minute should start your alarm bells.

Myocardial Infarction is a diagnosis made by ECG and cardiac enzyme (Troponin T) estimation. Clinically however the pain will be like angina but more severe, more crushing in nature and more prolonged. The pain will occur in the centre of the chest and radiate across to the shoulders and down the arms. The patient may become short of breath, cold and clammy, nauseous and have a weak pulse and blood pressure may fall.

The medical emergency team should be called immediately and GTN should be given followed by 300 mgs. aspirin crushed or chewed. Oxygen should be given at 15L/min and if consciousness is lost resuscitation as the ABCDE approach should be started.

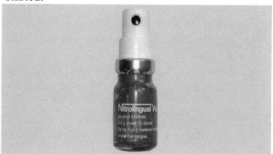

Glyceryl Trinitrate

27. <u>Resuscitation</u>

<u>Introduction</u>

Cardiopulmonary Resuscitation (CPR) consists of those procedures used to revive heart and lung function where they have ceased. Cardiopulmonary collapse has many causes but in most cases it will follow acute heart failure due to Myocardial Infarction ('heart attack'). There are situations where resuscitation would not be appropriate, such as when death is expected in someone very ill, where the attempt would be pointless, or where the patient has previously indicated that they do not wish to be resuscitated. For inpatients who fall into this category a Do Not Attempt Resuscitation (DNAR) form will have been completed; this is very unlikely for OMFS patients.

Myocardial Infarction (MI) is due to occlusive thrombus at the site of rupture or erosion of a plaque of atheroma in one of the coronary arteries. The process may take several hours and may be salvaged with clot dissolving drugs if they are administered early. Many

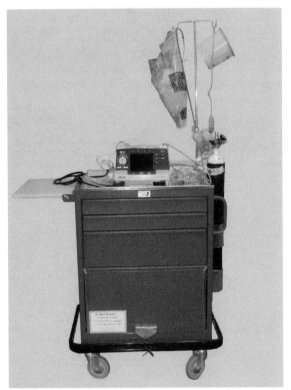

Resuscitation trolley. You can see an oxygen cylinder, intravenous fluids, a defibrillator and a sharps disposal bin.

patients will have the classic symptoms: crushing central chest pain radiating down the (usually) left arm, shortness of breath and collapse. However, it is possible to have a painless infarction, particularly in diabetics and the elderly; the patient may initially have just shortness of breath and then collapse. In the elderly it is possible to have a 'silent' Myocardial Infarction with no symptoms at all.

Infarction may be diagnosed with an ECG, but not necessarily. Usually diagnosis is retrospective, using serial ECG and blood levels of enzymes or proteins released from the cardiac muscle when damaged. Most useful is the titre of the cardiac proteins Troponin T and I. They are specific to cardiac muscle and are released within 4 to 6 hours of muscle death; they can remain elevated for up to two weeks.

The complications of MI vary, from immediate death due to acute heart failure, if a large part of the muscle infarcts, to none, if the infarct is small.

Arrhythmias can occur as a complication of MI, the commonest being ventricular fibrillation and ventricular tachycardia. These can be reversed with a direct current electric shock given with an Automatic External Defibrillator (AED). Pulseless Electrical Activity-PEA, (where the ECG shows a tracing but there is no contraction), or asystole (where there is no tracing at all), cannot be reversed with a shock.

Ventricular Fibrillation (VF) is rapid, irregular and un-coordinated electrical activity in the ventricles, probably due to re-entry circuits within localised areas of the myocardium. The ECG shows a coarse irregular waveform without discernible P, QRS or T waves. Effective contraction and cardiac output ceases, leading to loss of consciousness. It is often precipitated by ectopic beats or a burst of ventricular tachycardia, particularly when they are complications of acute MI. If it occurs within 48 hours of acute MI the prognosis is better than if it occurs later when more muscle damage has occurred. Ventricular fibrillation is the commonest cause of sudden death in the community.

The success rate for resuscitation of patients who 'arrest' is low. Fewer than a quarter of those who suffer a cardiac arrest in hospital survive to go home. The most likely to survive are those where the arrest is monitored and witnessed (as they would be in a coronary care

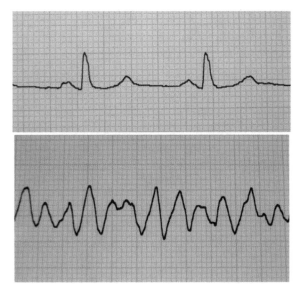

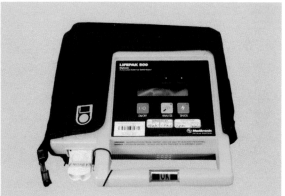

Automatic External Defibrillator (AED). This analyses the heart rhythm and advises you with audible instructions if the rhythm is 'shockable'.

Ventricular fibrillation (VF) on an ECG is obvious when compared to normal sinus rhythm at the top. This patient was being monitored on the coronary care unit when she went into VF after a myocardial infarction. Resuscitation was successful.

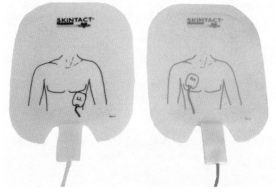

The two skin pads attached to the defibrillator have clear diagrams as to where they should be placed.

unit), where the arrest is caused by myocardial ischemia with an irritable myocardium, and where the patient is defibrillated immediately. In patients whose arrest occurs outside the coronary care unit in unmonitored areas it usually follows a slow progressive deterioration in their physiological well-being with hypoxemia and hypotension. This leads to asystole or a pulseless heart, in which case the prognosis is poor. Attempts have been made to avoid this by carrying out 'Early Warning Scores' in which a patient is awarded points on a scale depending on observation of respiratory rate, heart rate, blood pressure and level of consciousness. If a patient reaches a certain risk level then their nurse will call the critical care outreach team or medical emergency team, depending upon the local arrangements.

Resuscitation is divided into basic and advanced life support. Basic life support can be performed by a lay person who has been trained but who has no equipment other than perhaps a pocket airway to inflate the lungs from their own mouth.

Advanced life support requires equipment and specialised skills. In hospital there should be no such distinction; basic life support given by the first person to witness the collapse should continue seamlessly to defibrillation, if appropriate, and advanced

management by the medical emergency team who should have been summoned by calling 2222. After starting CPR you would normally expect the Emergency Team to arrive within a few minutes. However, modern automatic defibrillators will automatically analyse the electrical activity of the heart and decide if there is a 'shockable' rhythm, so you should get on with it and not wait for the team.

When a patient collapses after an MI their survival depends upon successful defibrillation with an AED. The sooner this is used the better their chance; each minute's delay reduces their chance by 10%. If they have just collapsed then they will have enough oxygen on board for a few minutes but you should still start with chest compression as this make ventricular fibrillation coarser and increases the chance of a successful defibrillation.

You will find there are numerous resuscitation

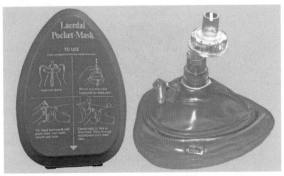

A pocket mask used for basic life support. The mask fits tightly around the mouth and nose to facilitate lung inflation without mouth contact. There is a filter on the end and a port to connect oxygen should it be available. There is guidance printed on the case.

trolleys containing all the necessary equipment throughout the hospital. This will be checked regularly and the defibrillator tested every morning. You should make sure you are familiar with the equipment.

The chances of you having to carry out CPR are low. This makes it important that you practise on a manikin at least once every six months and know the procedure by heart so that if needed you will be able to carry it out. Make sure to attend the resuscitation training sessions and get a certificate to prove that you have done it. CPR always gets tested in postgraduate

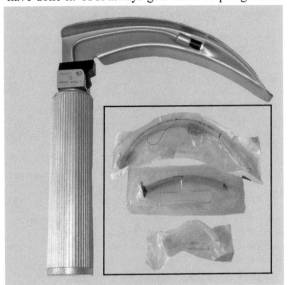

Airway management equipment is included on the resuscitation trolley. This includes the laryngoscope, endotracheal, nasopharyngeal and oral airways. You should only use the oral airway, leaving the use of the others to those trained in intubation.

dental examinations. This is a gift to the candidates as they all always do well, although a significant proportion do the chest compression too fast because they have not practised on a manikin recently.

Resuscitation procedure

The aim should be to start CPR immediately, and, if appropriate, defibrillate within three minutes at the most.

The following process is based on the Resuscitation Council's recommendations for in-hospital resuscitation and makes the following assumptions: the collapse has occurred during minor oral surgery and thus includes clearing the mouth of debris or obstruction; there are other health care professionals present who can participate in the process; there is certain equipment available which would not be available in a non-hospital setting such as ECG, pulse oximetry and blood pressure monitoring; there is a Medical Emergency Team or resuscitation team available to respond to a '2222' call; there are health care professionals present with the appropriate equipment and expertise to gain intra-venous access.

1. When you find a patient collapsed or witness a patient lose consciousness you should shout for help

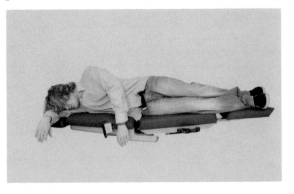

and check that there is nothing that will compromise your own personal safety.

2. You should shake the patient vigorously by the

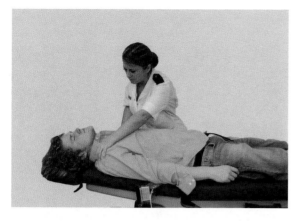

shoulders and shout, asking if they are OK, to see if there is any responsiveness. If patient is responsive, see box below:

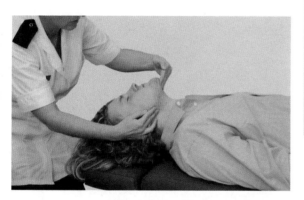

3. If no response turn patient on his back, open his airway by tilting his head back and lifting his chin forward.

If the patients is responsive at stage 2 or 5 above:

If it is a simple vaso-vagal syncope showing the signs described in previous chapter and the patient recovers quickly tip patient back, give oxygen and carry on.

Otherwise access the patient with ABCDE approach (below). Call medical emergency team as appropriate. Give patient oxygen trough mask and monitor with a pulse oximeter, attach ECG leads attach monitor and blood pressure cuffs and take readings. Gain venous access.

Hand over when medical emergency team arrive.

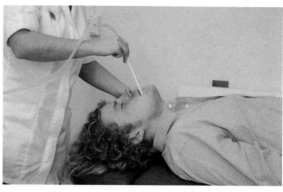

4. Check there is no obstruction in his mouth to compromise the airway; suck out if there is any debris.

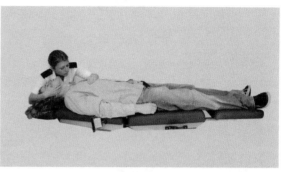

5. Listen for breathing and simultaneously look and feel for air and chest movement for 10 seconds (no longer). It is more reliable to check for respiration than attempting to feel for a pulse. If patient is responsive check carotid pulse and see box below:

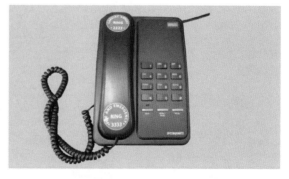

6. If there is no breathing obvious by 10 seconds ask your helper to call 'cardiac arrest' to the Medical Emergency Team by calling 2222. If you are still alone do it yourself.

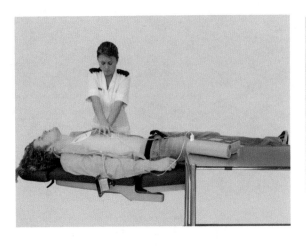

7. *Start CPR by compressing the chest in the middle of the lower half of the sternum for 4 - 5 cms (about $^1/_3$ its depth) 100 times per minute.*

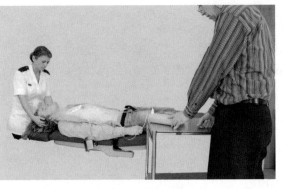

The AED, when ready, will instruct you to 'stand well clear of the patient' while it analyses the cardiac rhythm; it will tell you to shock the patient if it does not detect sinus rhythm and after further analysis of the electrical activity will tell you to start CPR again if appropriate. You should aim to defibrillate within 60 to 120 seconds; every minute's delay reduces the chance of a successful outcome by about 10%.

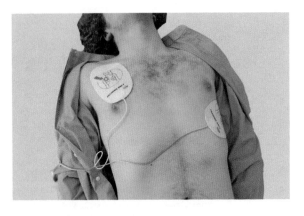

8. *Put on the Automatic External Defibrillator (AED) pads in the positions shown on the pads. Do this without interrupting chest compression.*

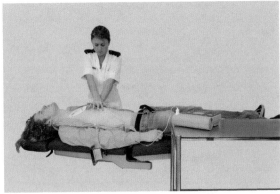

10. *If the patient does not respond, and the AED tells you to, restart CPR with chest compression.*

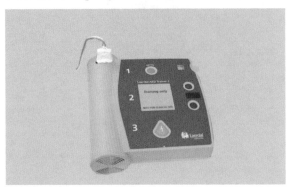

9. *Plug the lead into the AED, press the on switch and follow the verbal instructions.*

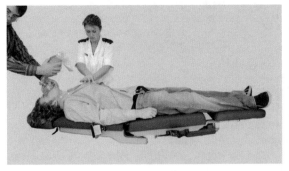

11. *Now introduce ventilation using the face mask with a reservoir bag. You can place an oral airway to prevent tongue obstruction. The lungs should be*

ventilated with the bag over the airway for 1 second with enough volume to expand the chest as seen in normal breathing. Oxygen should be attached to the bag as soon as possible. Chest compression and ventilation should proceed at the ratio of 30:2. Chest compression is the more important.

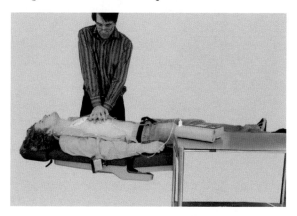

12. Change the person doing chest compression every 2 minutes to prevent fatigue. The AED will analyse the rhythm periodically and tell you to shock the patient if necessary. If you have sufficient helpers someone can place an IV line before the Medical Emergency Team arrive.

Resuscitation in examinations

For examinations you should memorise the resuscitation council's recommendations for dental practice.

This assumes no IV access skills and no expertise in feeling a carotid pulse and no on site emergency team. It relies on you calling 999 for back up.

You should practise on a manikin, in particular the rate of cardiac compression which candidates often get too fast. You should practise lung inflation with mouth inflation and a pocket mask which is easier to get an oral air seal with than a bag and mask.

In the exam you will have to operate alone which means you will need to simulate calling for help (including dialling 999) and fetching equipment yourself before starting chest compression.

The principle is that unless you can defibrillate the patient with the automatic external defibrillator the patient will die.

ABCDE of assessment of collapsed patient

The process gives a structured approach to assessment. It starts with the easiest to recognise, and most dangerous, problems which are easier to deal with and progresses to the more difficult.

A - Airway
Upper airway obstruction. If they can answer a verbal question then they are not obstructed. Caused by secretions or vomit or swelling. Tongue may be fallen back if patient not fully conscious. Stridor (wheezing on breathing out) is a sign. Lift the chin, tilt head, suction. May need anaesthetist if upper airway is obstructed.

B - Breathing
Respiratory rate is most important. Look for chest expansion, depth of breath & use of accessory muscle of respiration. Listen for wheeze from end of bed, then with stethoscope. What is their colour: are they pale or blue? Feel if the chest is expanding equally. Give them a short spell of 15L/ min. of O_2. Their saturation on pulse oximeter must be 90% at the very least.

C - Circulation
Look for pallor, anaemia or signs of blood loss. Check capillary refill time (normally < 2 secs). Feel central (carotid) pulse; if absent systolic probably <70. Feel peripheral limb temperature and peripheral pulse; if no radial pulse systolic <90. Check pulse rate & rhythm. (BP may be normal in severe hypovolaemia shock.) What is the O2 saturation & urine output? Both may be low in hypovolaemia or cardiogenic shock. If not obvious sign of heart failure assume hypovolaemia and give 200 mls fluid then reassess.

D - Disability (Neurological)
Are they conscious, alert and orientated and conversing or confused? State can be described according to the A V P U system. A – alert, V – responds to voice, P – responds to pain, U – unresponsive. Can use Glasgow Coma Scale to describe patient's condition . Measure blood glucose and nurse in supine position if unconscious.

E - Exposure (for full examination)
Expose the patient to carry out a full physical examination in more detail.

28. <u>Examination of Cardiovascular and Respiratory Systems</u>

In this chapter we will introduce the basis of the medical clerking and the examination process and consider important cardiovascular and respiratory pathology seen in surgical patients. We will briefly remind you of the basic pathology which is likely to produce physical signs in the cardiovascular and respiratory systems.

All patients coming into hospital for operation, either as a day-case or with an overnight stay, should have an assessment made of their cardiovascular and respiratory systems. Traditionally, the patient was "clerked" by a house officer on the ward. This involved a full history, examination and investigations such as blood tests, a chest radiograph and ECG. This has largely been superseded by dedicated nurse-led pre-operative assessment clinics.

Although every patient receiving anaesthetic will be seen pre-operatively by an anaesthetist, who will go through their medical history and examine as necessary, it is still a useful exercise for OMFS trainees to clerk and examine inpatients to help appreciate systemic disease and how it may affect surgery and anaesthesia.

It should also be noted that as an OMFS trainee you will be assisting in the management of post-operative patients on the ward. The post-operative period is critical; occasionally these patients develop medical complications rather than complications from the actual surgery itself. In order to hand over to your senior colleagues, it will be helpful if you are able to understand what might be happening and form a rough differential diagnosis.

It is important to realise that the medical history is the most important part of eliciting disease; physical examination usually helps confirm what has already been discovered during history taking. The full medical clerking also includes examination of the gastrointestinal, renal, urinary, neurological and locomotor systems which we will not address as they are usually not significant in most OMFS patients.

Possibly the most important part of the examination will be the blood pressure. Hypertension is a risk factor for cardiovascular disease especially heart failure, ischaemic heart disease, strokes and peripheral vascular disease as well as chronic kidney disease. You cannot expect to be able to elicit all physical signs with a few months' practice but you may expect to be able to pick up the main ones associated with severe cardiovascular and respiratory disease.

<u>Important cardiovascular and respiratory pathology</u>

A basic knowledge of common and serious cardiovascular and respiratory pathology will aid in putting clinical signs found on examination into context.

Heart failure is when the heart is having difficulty pumping blood (and therefore oxygen and nutrients) to the peripheral tissues. There are numerous possible causes of failure. Most commonly it will result from myocardial ischaemia, hypertension, arrhythmias (often secondary to ischemia), valve disease, metabolic diseases such as diabetes or thyroid disease or any disease process which damages the cardiac muscle (myopathy). Sometimes failure may result from lung disease; chronic obstructive pulmonary disease (COPD) can result in pulmonary hypertension causing heart failure ("cor pulmonale").

The most common cause is ischaemic heart disease (IHD) where, through a lack of oxygen, the muscle of the myocardium has suffered irreversible damage and is no longer able to pump adequately. Most patients will give a history of angina, report a previous myocardial infarction or will have undergone angioplasty. Signs of IHD can also be found in some ECGs, which are beyond the scope of this book.

In some cases the heart may fail as a result of a rhythm disorder (arrhythmias) secondary to IHD or old age; this is diagnosed by ECG. Atrial fibrillation (AF) is the most common rhythm abnormality causing heart failure. AF is diagnosed by feeling the peripheral pulse as "irregularly irregular".

Valvular heart disease can cause heart failure, when a valve is either incompetent (incomplete closure of a valve causes retrograde flow) or stenosed (a stiff or thickened valve resists smooth anterograde flow). These may be suspected when an added heart sound or "murmur" may be heard on auscultation of the heart.

In mild heart failure the patient may have no symptoms at rest but on exertion the diseased heart may not be able to pump efficiently enough to provide adequate tissue oxygenation. This may result in shortness of breath on exertion.

The signs of heart failure can be more easily understood if one divides the pumping heart into two sides. The right side receives deoxygenated blood from the peripheral tissues and pumps this to the lungs. The left side receives oxygenated blood from the lungs and pumps this to the peripheral tissues. Blood restricted from efficient entry through a failing right side of the heart will lead to increased central venous pressure and fluid accumulation in the peripheries; this is seen clinically as a raised jugular venous pressure (JVP) and ankle, leg or sacral pitting oedema. Blood damming behind a failing left side of heart accumulates in the lungs causing pulmonary oedema, (producing shortness of breath) and in severe cases pleural effusions. This is detected clinically as basal crepitations on auscultation and dullness to percussion at the lung bases.

The most common respiratory disease you are likely to encounter is an upper respiratory tract infection (URTI). This is a relative contraindication to having general anaesthetic as patients are more likely to have laryngo-bronchospasm with an endotracheal tube and there is increased risk of pneumonia. Although it is sensible to delay surgery until at least two weeks after recovery, complications can, to a certain extent, be anticipated. Thus it is prudent to continue with urgent surgery and delay non-urgent cases.

Asthma is the most common co-existing chronic respiratory disease you are most likely to come across pre-operatively in young patients. Usually this is mild and patients will have the symptoms of wheezing or coughing only when they have a cold, and are controlled with a salbutamol +/- corticosteroid inhaler. These patients are quite easily managed by the anaesthetist.

Patients with more severe asthma may give a history of requiring previous hospital admissions or home nebuliser therapy. A nebuliser is a much more efficient and effective mechanism of delivering inhaled medication than inhalers. These patients may need a short course of prednisolone to prevent an acute attack and monitoring with a peak expiratory flow meter. Clinical signs on examination may include dyspnoea and wheeze during an attack, but otherwise would be expected to be normal.

Chronic obstructive pulmonary disease (COPD), unlike asthma, is largely irreversible airways constriction. It is commoner in older patients and is almost always associated with cigarette smoking. COPD patients exist on a spectrum where mild sufferers only develop shortness of breath on exertion, whereas in severe cases patients require long-term oxygen therapy and nebulisers at home. Like asthmatics, they are likely to be on regular inhalers. Severe COPD patients will likely not be candidates for surgery under general anaesthetic unless for trauma or cancer. If you suspect that a patient is having an acute attack of asthma or COPD, seek help from medical colleagues as these patients may require oxygen, nebulisers and corticosteroids.

Many of the abnormal physical signs seen in respiratory disease are common to some of those found in cardiovascular disease so it is sensible to develop a sequence that you become comfortable with to examine both systems together.

Equipment for examination of the cardiovascular and respiratory systems

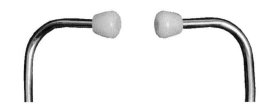

The earpiece of the stethoscope should fit comfortably in the ears, facing forward.

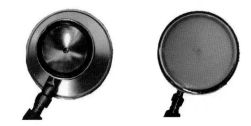

Both the bell and the diaphragm of the stethoscope should be used. The bell, pressed lightly on the chest wall, is best for hearing low pitched sounds, whereas the diaphragm is best used for high frequency sounds and is therefore used more frequently.

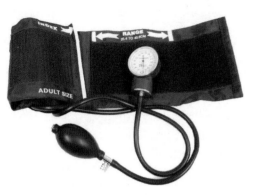

The aneroid sphygmomanometer replaced the mercury manometer for recording blood pressure. Like the mercury sphygmomanometer it requires the use of the stethoscope for listening to the sounds at the brachial artery.

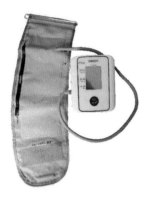

Mostly we now use a digital machine to record BP. This detects oscillation of the blood and does not require a stethoscope.

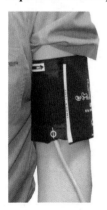 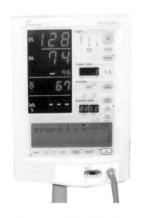

Most wards and clinics will use a digital device such as this Dynamap machine. It also records pulse rate.

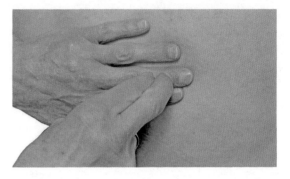

To elicit a chest dullness percuss by placing the middle finger of the left hand flush with the chest wall and, with the end of the right middle finger, hit it twice on the middle phalanx in quick succession, at right angles using wrist movement.

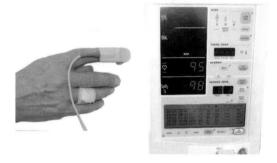

Pulse oximetry. The sensor is attached to the finger. The Pulse rate on the 'datascope' monitor (right) is 95 and PO2 is 98 %

The examination process

A full medical clerking will include examination of the cardio-vascular, respiratory, gastro-intestinal, neurological, urinary and locomotor systems. We will only include the cardio-vascular and respiratory systems as generally these will be important in assessment of fitness for surgery.

The general scheme of the examination involves initially observing the patient at the bedside, then starting at the hands, moving to the arm, face, neck, chest, abdomen and finishing at the feet.

Initially

Wash your hands, introduce yourself to the patient ask permission to examine them, ask if they have any pain anywhere, expose them from the waist upwards and reposition them supine and at 45 degrees.

General Inspection

Note their general appearance: do they look unwell, uncomfortable, in pain, pale or clammy? Do they have dyspnoea (shortness of breath)? Observe their rate of breathing: are their lips pursed on breathing out producing a prolonged expiratory phase; are they using their accessory muscles of respiration? Observe their lips for cyanosis and conjunctiva for the paleness of anaemia.

Ask about pain as you do not want to cause more pain by examining them. Dyspnoea could be caused by respiratory disease or heart failure. Note that impairment of blood oxygen would have to be very severe before central cyanosis would be visible in the lips (at least 5g/dL of deoxygenated haemoglobin in the peripheral blood). Central cyanosis is best observed on the lips/tongue (centrally), as peripheral cyanosis seen on the fingertips can also be seen in Raynaud's phenomenon and in cold weather. Anaemia would need to be severe to be observed clinically as pallor. Normal respiratory rate is 12 - 16 breaths per minute. Breathing out slowly through pursed lips occurs in airway disease and subconsciously helps keep the airways open to the end of the respiratory cycle to aid gas exchange. Use of accessory muscles indicates difficulty. The chest may move asymmetrically in certain lung diseases.

Hands

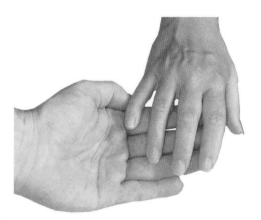

Examine for nicotine staining, warmth and clubbing.

Nicotine staining indicates long-term cigarette smoking and is a risk factor for cardiovascular and respiratory disease. A patient with severe pulmonary disease may have CO_2 retention which causes dilated peripheral veins and warm extremities. In very severe disease there may be peripheral cyanosis. Clubbing is enlargement of the terminal end of the finger over the distal phalanx; the nails may be curved both horizontally and longitudinally. Clubbing can be congenital as in cyanotic heart disease or acquired as in endocarditis, chronic hypoxia, bronchogenic carcinoma, mesothelioma, interstitial lung disease, as well as certain gastrointestinal disease such as inflammatory bowel disease and liver disease. However in many cases clubbing is not associated with any underlying pathology.

Examine the radial pulse

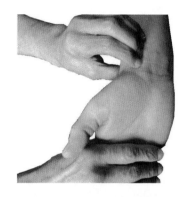

Use the tips of two fingers to palpate the radial artery. Observe and record if the pulse is 'full' or weak, regular or irregular. Count the beats per minute, time over 15 seconds and multiply by 4.

The commonest irregularities are extra systoles which may occur regularly, or atrial fibrillation which always gives an irregular irregularity. These are indications for an ECG for more accurate diagnosis. The normal pulse rate is between 60 and 100 beats per minute with an average of 72 beats at rest. Even mild exercise or emotion will raise it. It will be higher in children, perhaps between 90 and 110, and lower in the elderly, 55 to 60. Well trained athletes may have a low resting rate.

Record the blood pressure

This can be measured manually using the aneroid sphygmomanometer and stethoscope or digitally using automatic machines (as below). You should ensure you are proficient using manual methods before becoming overly reliant on nurses' readings.

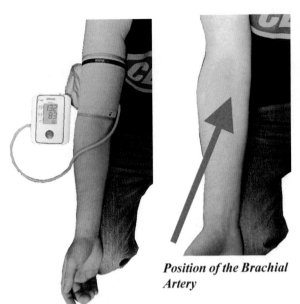

Position of the Brachial Artery

The sphygmomanometer cuff should fit snugly around the arm about 2cm above the ante-cubital space. Recline the patient comfortably. Palpate the brachial artery, then place the cuff with the arrow which is marked on the cuff approximating to the position of the artery. The cuff should be placed at the level of the heart. Palpate the radial pulse and inflate the cuff to 30 mmHg above the level at which the radial pulse disappears. If using and aneroid sphygmomanometer. place the stethoscope diaphragm over the artery and release the pressure slowly. Listen through the stethoscope carefully; the Korotkov sounds are heard as the blood passes through the artery. At first these are faint and tapping and then a swishing quality is noted. The sounds intensify as the pressure falls, and become muffled, then disappear. The systolic pressure is when the sounds are first heard, and the diastolic pressure is recorded when the sounds disappear.

If using a digital machine you will not need the stethoscope , it will record the pressure automatically based on blood oscillation.

A reading above 140/90 should be repeated. If this occurs over three occasions the GP should be informed so they can monitor and treat if necessary. If over 160/110 the anaesthetist may want to postpone a routine case until it is controlled. The risk of hypertension causing an adverse cardiovascular event during anaesthesia is not quantified, but should such an event occur no one would wish to feel responsible. It is important that all adults have their blood pressure measured intermittently. Hypertension is associated with a shortened life span due to its numerous complications. Atheroma formation is accelerated by hypertension so there is an increased risk of ischaemic heart disease, peripheral vascular disease, aneurysm and strokes. If severe it can cause myocardial hypertrophy and pulmonary venous congestion. It may affect the small vessels of the cerebral and renal circulation.

Inspect and palpate the chest

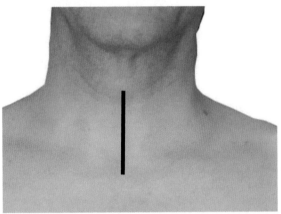

Observe and palpate the trachea (marked with black line) to see if it is central or deviated to either side. Observe for any deformity of the chest wall and that both sides expand equally during inspiration. Note any scars from previous surgery.

A trachea deviated from the midline is abnormal. The trachea may be deviated away from the side of a tension pneumothorax or large plural effusion or towards a lung which is collapsed, severely fibrosed or infiltrated with tumour. Movement of the chest wall may be reduced in certain pulmonary conditions e.g. consolidation. Certain chest deformities such as a barrel shaped chest suggest hyperinflation as may occur in COPD. Reduced lung expansion unilaterally may be due to lung collapse, pleural effusion or pneumothorax or bilateral in lung fibrosis.

Examine the Jugular Venous Pressure (JVP)

Recline the patient at 45° and ask them to look at a fixed point on their left. The jugular venous pressure is normally 5 cms above the left atrium which is about 5cms below the manubrial sternal angle (arrow A). Put a finger across the external jugular at the base of the neck and press gently. A column of blood will become visible in the vein (arrow B), which will flow

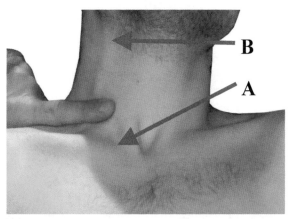

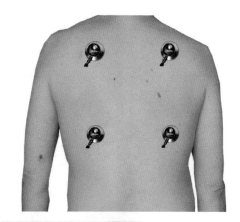

away when the finger is removed. In heart failure the column may be there without the external pressure. The JVP will be the height of any column of blood visible in the Internal Jugular Vein + 5 cms above the manubrial sternal angle (arrow A).

The JVP is a rough approximation of the Central Venous Pressure (CVP) which will be increased in heart failure and decreased in hypovolaemia (significant blood loss). In a patient acutely ill with severe haemodynamic upset (or potentially so, such as in major surgery) this may be measured with a central CVP line and manometer. A specific measurement, as described above, is probably too ambitious. It will usually be enough to say that the JVP is raised if the column of blood is anything other than not visible or just visible at the base of the neck.

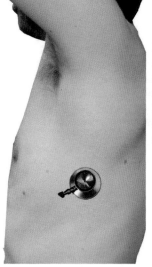

You should likewise examine beneath the axilla on the left for the middle lobe of the lung, there is no middle lobe on the right.

Auscultate and percuss the chest

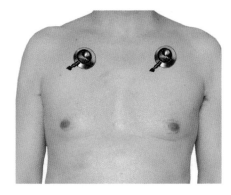

Auscultate with the diaphragm of the stethoscope and percuss the upper lobes at the front and upper and lower lobes at the back.

You should particularly examine the lung bases; ask the patient to lean forward and cough. Auscultate the base of the lung field for crepitations. These will sound like rustling tissue paper. Percussion of the basal lung fields may produce a dull note if there is a pleural effusion due to severe heart failure. A dull note will be heard in inflammation such as pneumonia. A hyper-resonant note may also be heard in pneumothorax or chronically where the lungs are hyper-inflated in COPD or asthma.

Normal breath sounds are described as vesicular. A wheeze may be heard in asthma, and crackles may be heard in upper respiratory tract infection. Bronchial breathing is a harsh sound of air passing through the trachea and large airways. It may be heard over the peripheral lung fields if they are consolidated such as in pneumonia; this is because the sound will be conducted more efficiently. Get into the habit of going through these steps in a methodical way; it will only take seconds when you are familiar with it. However, for a surgical clerking there is no need to write down long lists of negative findings. Become familiar with the percussion note heard over normal lung which is resonant. Become familiar with the normal vesicular breath sounds.

Palpate for the heart

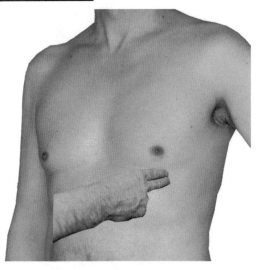

Palpate for the apex beat which should normally be at the 5th intercostal space in the mid clavicular line. Note the position of the apex and whether there is a 'thrill' which is a palpable murmur and best felt with a flat palm held horizontally across the 2nd and 5th intercostal spaces in the mid clavicular line.

Normally you should palpate with the flat of your hand to find the apex and then when located palpate more precisely with two fingers, as shown.

The position of the apex beat may be displaced down and laterally if the left ventricle is hypertrophied as may occur in valve disease or severe hypertension.

Listen for murmurs

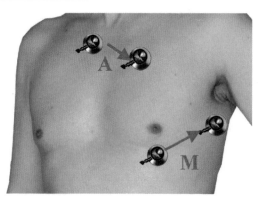

Mitral murmurs. (Area M) Listen at the 5th inter costal space (just beneath the left nipple) in the mid clavicle line. This is the mitral area (M) which extends from the apex to the mid axillary line. Mitral murmurs are often low pitched and 'rumbling'; they are best heard with the bell of the stethoscope. First listen with the patient sitting up, and holding his breath in full expiration. However, a quiet mitral murmur will best be heard with the patient lying on their left side in full expiration which brings the heart over towards the chest wall. While listening collate the findings with the cardiac cycle by palpating the carotid artery pulse. Aortic murmurs (Area A) tend to be more high pitched and are heard with the diaphragm of the stethoscope from the right of the sternum at the level of the first rib, passing over to the right of the sternum and down to the second intercostal space.

You will not become proficient in recognising different types of murmur but try to become comfortable about recognising the normal heart sounds and telling if a murmur is present. If you detect one it would be a bonus to differentiate between systolic and diastolic by feeling the carotid pulse as you listen. All diastolic murmurs are abnormal but a systolic murmur may be an innocent 'flow' murmur if heard in very fit young adults or children; otherwise systolic murmurs are usually due to aortic valve stenosis (common in the elderly) or mitral valve regurgitation. If you think you hear a murmur tell the anaesthetist. The patient will probably need an ECHO cardiogram and referral for a cardiology opinion.

Examine the abdomen

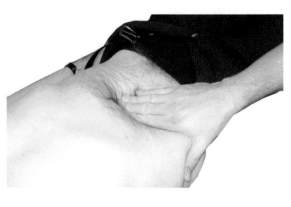

Palpate the abdomen with the patient lying flat with arms laid by his side. Stoop or kneel to his level and gently palpate the abdomen with the flat of the hand from the right iliac fossa to the right costal margin.

An engorged liver from heart failure will be tender, smoothly enlarged and palpable below the left costal margin. A normal liver should not be palpable. In severe heart failure fluid may enter the peritoneal cavity (ascites). A large aortic aneurysm may be palpated by feeling centrally in the abdomen. It will expand in size with each heart beat.

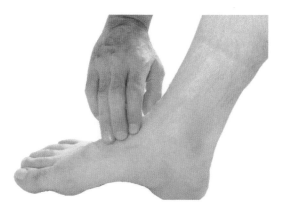

Examine the feet

Feel for the dorsalis pedis pulse which will be weak or absent in peripheral vascular disease. Examine for oedema consequent upon right sided heart failure. This will show 'pitting' if you push your thumb into it.

In heart failure fluid will accumulate in and around the systemic circulation. This will lead to an increased central venous pressure and hence JVP (see before), swelling of the feet or ankles and a smoothly enlarged tender liver (below). If the patient is bed bound the fluid may accumulate in the sacral area rather than the feet. Atheromatous disease in the arteries may produce ischaemic heart disease, cerebrovascular accidents (strokes and transient ischaemic attacks), aneurysms and peripheral vascular disease. The latter may show as weak or absent pulses, cold feet, ulcers or gangrene. The dorsalis pedis pulse is felt in the first metatarsal space. Alternative is the posterior tibial artery midway between the medial malleolus (ankle) and the heel.

An example of what to write.

Date

Mr Cedrick Booth   73 ♂

Retired barber

History

Past Medical History

Medication

Social History

O/E °anaemia °cyanosis °SOB

　　°clubbing

P=　76/min reg

BP = 120/85 JVP ®

Trachea　　　　RR 12/min

Expansion=　　Apex ®

HS I & II + O

PNR　　　BS vesicular

°oedema　　　PPV

Abdomen soft　°organomegaly

Date

Patients Name   Age Sex

Occupation

History of presenting complaint

Past Medical History

Medication

Social History

On examination . No anaemia, cyanosis, shortness of breath or clubbing

Pulse 76 per minute, regular

Blood pressure 120 systolic 85 diastolic

Jugular venous pressure not raised

Trachea central respiratory rate 12 per minute

Lung expansion equal, apex beat not displaced

Heart sounds 1 & 2 heard with no added sounds

Percussion note resonant, breath sounds vesicular

No peripheral oedema, peripheral pulse present.

Abdomen soft, no organ enlargement (part liver)

Other Shorthand

Apex ↘　　　　*Apex beat displaced down and laterally*

HS I ⌐∿∼II　　*Murmur heard between heart sounds 1 & 2 i.e. systolic*

HS I ⸺ II ∿　*Murmur after sound 2 i.e. diastolic*

94

29. <u>The Sterile Supply Service</u>

Nearly all instruments used in surgery will come on trays or in baskets double wrapped and autoclaved. Bench top sterilizers, such as those frequently used in dental practices, are not used in hospitals because of their unreliability and the need for vigorous and documented daily testing and servicing. Some instruments which are infrequently used will be packed singly, and some will be single use and disposable. The instruments are used directly from the trays or baskets and are sent back to sterile supply in them. Some items cannot be adequately cleaned prior to sterilization so should be treated as single use; surgical burs fall into this category. Before being returned, gross contamination should be removed from instruments whilst wearing kitchen gloves.

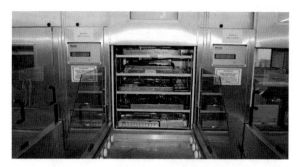

They do not leave their tray or basket which is loaded into racks and put into the washer/disinfector machine. The instruments are not subjected to any manual cleaning but are processed through the machine where they are mechanically cleaned with jets of water at 90°C in an alkaline detergent, then dried.

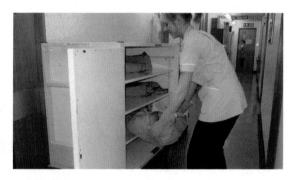

Dirty instruments are returned for processing in wheeled strong metal trolleys.

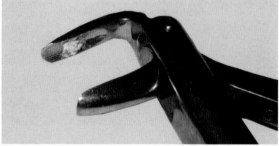

This pair of extraction forceps has gone through the whole process and retains compacted dentine on its beaks; it cannot be sterile. Gross contaminants should have been removed in the clinic prior to sending for processing and if not should have been noticed at the later visual inspection.

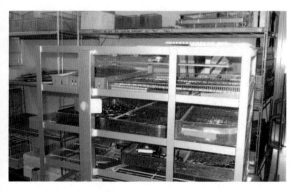

On arrival the instruments are unwrapped and placed into racks in the holding bay.

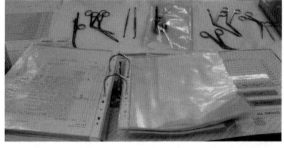

The now clean and dry instruments, trays and baskets are inspected to ensure that the instruments are visibly clean, are not damaged and are all present when checked against the instrument list for each tray.

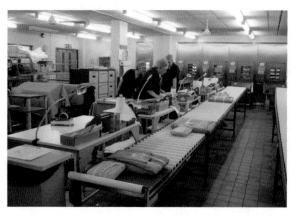

They pass along a conveyor and are double wrapped.

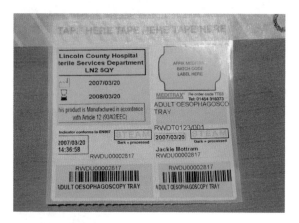

A label which contains bar codes is placed. These codes identify the hospital, the type of tray and the number of the individual tray.

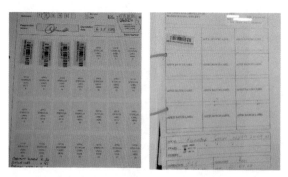

These bar codes are later used for the log of the trays which have been autoclaved in the department (left) and also in the individual patient's notes (right) so that the instruments used on each individual patient can be identified in the future.

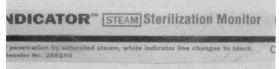

Each tray has a sterilization monitor indicator packed within it. The bar is sensitive to the steam, temperature and time. When the tray is finally opened for use if the bar is not black then it has not been processed sufficiently to guarantee sterility.

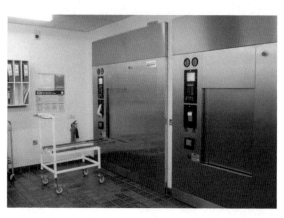

The packed trays are then processed through the autoclave itself. This vacuum autoclave draws all the air out and then injects steam under pressure. It repeats this alternately four times and on the last occasion it holds the steam in at between 134 and 137° for 3 to 3½ minutes at 2 bar pressure. The trays are then dried. The whole cycle takes 45 minutes.

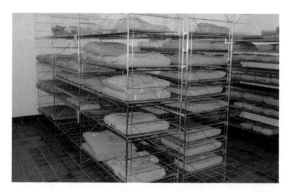

The trays are then stored for distribution to the operating theatres, wards and clinics. They are good for about a year.

30. <u>Surgical Instruments</u>

You will already be familiar with the common instruments used for dental extractions. This chapter seeks to introduce you to some more of the instruments used in OMFS that you are likely to come across. Many of these are named after surgical or dental characters of former years who designed them, or sometimes simply after those who used them or made them popular.

Surgical instruments are usually supplied for use in pre packed trays of instruments commonly used together. Those used less often may be individually packed. The nurses in the operating theatre will keep a card index of which trays and individual instruments are needed by particular surgeons for particular operations. For surgery in the outpatient clinic there are minor oral surgery sets, which contain basic instruments for exodontia, and soft tissue sets, which contain the fewer instruments needed for biopsies and skin surgery. In the operating theatre there will be oral surgery sets, facial trauma, osteotomy, plating sets and 'wiring of jaw' sets which are nowadays infrequently used.

Each pre-packed tray of instruments comes from the Central Sterile Supply Department and is double wrapped in sterile drapes and closed with autoclave tape. The trays are designed to sit on disinfected stainless steel wheeled trolleys. Infrequently used instruments will be double wrapped, and designed for a nurse to open the outer layer and drop the instrument wrapped within an inner layer onto the sterile tray already opened.

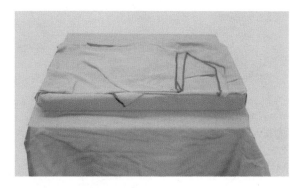

The inner of the two drapes is opened after the nurse has donned sterile gloves.

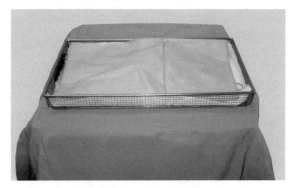

The tray contains sterile (green) drapes to cover the patient, in this case for minor oral surgery. One goes behind the patient's head and the other over them.

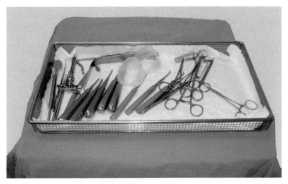

The instruments are arranged in the approximate order they are to be used. The nurse arranges them tidily, with the most used ones on the sterile drape outside the tray.

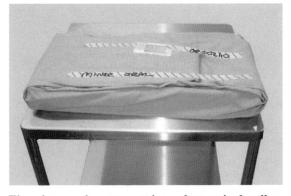

The minor oral surgery set is on the surgical trolley. The first layer of the drape is opened with clean hands touching only the outside and is allowed to drop back around the trolley. Thus:

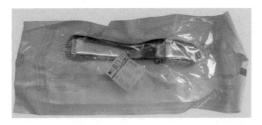

Individually packed retractor. The wrapping is designed to be peeled open and dropped onto a sterile tray.

Instruments used chiefly for Minor Oral Surgery

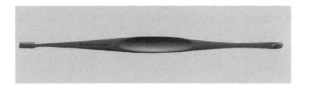

Howarth's[1] nasal raspatory. Used as a retractor and periosteal elevator for raising muco-periosteal flaps.

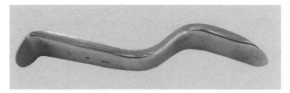

Minnesota retractor. Probably the most useful instrument for retracting muco-periosteal flaps whilst drilling bone.

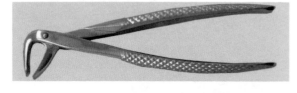

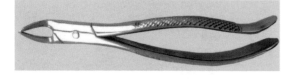

Upper and lower premolar dental extraction forceps are usually provided. They are suitable for most extractions. If any others are required they are packed separately and individually.

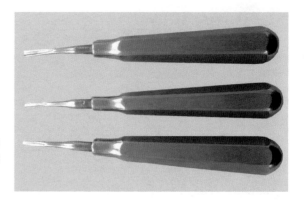

Coupland's[2] chisels are the most used dental elevators, size 1 to 3. They can be used to split teeth that have been partly divided with a bur, and to elevate teeth and roots. Size 1 is placed between bone and tooth and rotated to move the tooth remnant into space created with a bur. Only when some movement has been achieved should a larger size be used. They should never be used like a lever.

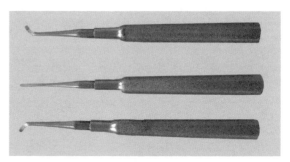

Warwick James[3] elevators are the next most useful. There is a straight one and there are two curved, left and right. They are used for elevating small fragments of dental roots.

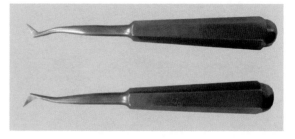

Cryer's[4] elevators, left and right, are used to elevate the remaining single root of double rooted teeth and buccally placed upper third molars.

¹ *Walter Goldie Howarth (1879 - 1962) was an ENT surgeon, who qualified at Cambridge in 1905 and later studied otolaryngology in Vienna & Berlin. He became the first Rhino laryngologist at St Thomas's Hospital. His instrument was devised for use in ENT surgery but is favoured by OMFS surgeons as well as being used in other surgical crafts.*

²*Douglas Charles William Coupland (1901 –1936) qualified as a dentist from Toronto in 1922. He studied exodontia at the Mayo Clinic and then practised oral surgery in Ottawa. He developed his chisels/gouges during the 1920s. They were initially produced in sets of 8 or 12, later reduced to 3.*

³*William Warwick James (1874-1965) was medically & dentally qualified, worked in dental practice as well as on the staff of the Royal Dental, the Middlesex and Great Ormond Street Hospitals. He took a scientific interest in dental development, the pathology of caries and periodontal disease. He wrote many books and papers, continuing well after his retirement. He fought in the First World War in France and later treated facial injuries sustained in the war. He kept all the clinical records, which resulted in a book in the 1950s. A member of the Zoological Society, he wrote about comparative anatomy of the teeth and jaws. He established a research fellowship at the Royal Dental Hospital and devised a technique for removing third molars by taking out lingual bone with a chisel. This was the forerunner of the now almost obsolete lingual split technique.*

⁴*Matthew H Cryer (1840-1921) was born in Manchester, but emigrated to the USA when he was aged 9. He became dentally and medically qualified and was appointed Professor of Oral Surgery in Pennsylvania in 1897. He designed extraction forceps and elevators.*

⁵*Cyril Bowdler Henry (1893 - 1981) qualified in dentistry in 1915 and medicine in 1919. He worked in private practice in Harley Street and consulted at the Westminster and Royal Dental Hospitals. He researched into and promoted the prophylactic removal of developing third molars and diathermy in dentistry. He was one of the first surgeons in the UK to carry out osteotomies for jaw deformity. An enthusiastic supporter of dual dental and medical qualification, he donated £10,000 to the Royal College of Surgeons for a scholarship to aid young dentists or doctors to gain a second qualification.*

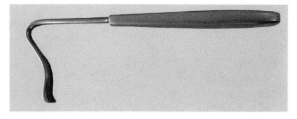

Bowdler-Henry⁵ rake retractor. Used to retract mucoperiosteal flaps during exodontia.

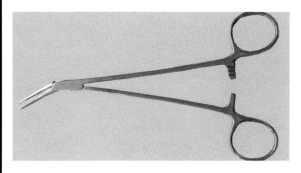

Fickling's⁶ forceps. Used to retrieve loose matter from the mouth, it has a toothed end.

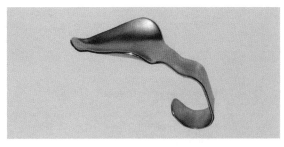

Laster upper third molar retractor. The pointed end is inserted beneath a muco-periosteal flap behind the maxillary tuberosity while the cheek is retracted to give a good visualisation. This gives excellent access for using a chisel or otherwise, and allows the tooth to be elevated with little risk of backwards displacement into the infra temporal fossa.

⁶ *Ben Fickling (1909 - 2007) studied dentistry & medicine concurrently. He was one of the dentists who teamed up with plastic surgeons to treat maxillofacial war injuries. He worked with Rainsford Mowlem at Hill End Hospital, St Albans. He co authored 'Injuries of the Jaws and Face' with Kelsey Fry and collaborated in the design of the box frame for the fixation of facial fractures. He was a founding member of the British Association of Oral Surgeons.*

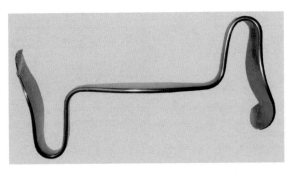

Ward's[1] third molar retractor. The blade fits under buccal muco-periosteal flap at the angle of the mouth and gives excellent exposure of the third molar area. We still use it for those occasions when wisdom teeth are removed under anaesthetic, for mandibular osteotomies and when plating fractures at the angle.

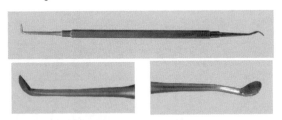

Ward's periosteal elevator

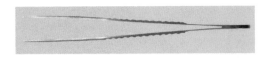

Mitchell's[2] trimmer. Used as a curette.

Instruments used chiefly for soft tissue surgery

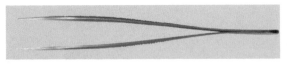

Gillies's[3] forceps. Used to approximate wound ends while suturing. There is a toothed version which grips firmly and non toothed version which is kinder to the tissues.

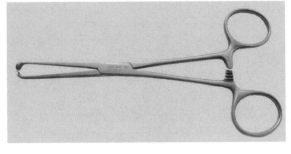

Adson's toothed forceps. Slightly smaller than the Gillies and more suitable for fine work. Alfred Washington Adson (1887—1951)

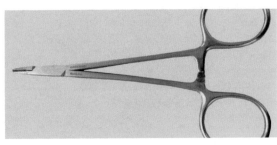

Crile[4] -Wood needle holders. For suturing.

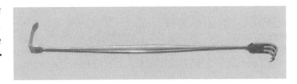

Kilner's[5] 'Cats paw' retractor

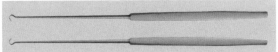

Gillies skin hooks. Used as a pair to approximate the edges of a skin wound whilst suturing.

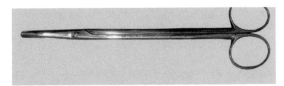

McIndoe[6] scissors. Larger scissors for dissecting soft tissues.

Allis[7] forceps. For holding soft tissues usually under some tension while being removed. .

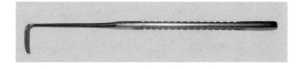

Langenbeck[8] retractor. Available in several sizes, it is used to retract the edges of a wound while dissecting beneath.

[1]*Sir Terence Ward (1906 - 1991) started his career in dentistry as apprentice to a dental mechanic and progressed via degrees in dentistry and medicine to become a founding member of the Faculty of Dental Surgery of the Royal College of Surgeons of England (and later its Dean) and the first President of the British Association of Oral Surgeons. During the Second World War he became involved at East Grinstead in treating facial injuries of RAF crew, with Sir Archibald McIndoe, and later he was appointed as the head of the OMFS service where he established a department which has trained many OMFS Surgeons.*

[2]*William Mitchell (1854-1914) trained in Michigan before moving to London where he became a General Dental Practitioner. Mitchell invented many instruments but none as popular as his 'trimmer' which has many uses but which was probably intended to trim the cemento-enamel junction after crown preparation. (Dattani A. & Hayes S. J. Br. Dent. J. 2015; 219: 459-461)*

[3]*Sir Harold Gillis (1882 - 1960) was a New Zealander. He was trained as an Otolaryngologist but developed many techniques of plastic surgery. In France during the First World War he worked with a dentist who was treating jaw injuries, and was inspired by the work. Eventually in England he developed the specialist facial injury unit at Queens Hospital, Sidcup. He had a large private practice between the two world wars but during the second he continued his treatment of injuries at Rooksdown House, Basingstoke. There are many techniques and instruments associated with Gillies's name and he is widely considered to be the father of modern plastic surgery.*

[4]*George Washington Crile (1864 - 1943) was in the premier league of innovative surgeons. He practised in Cleveland, Ohio. He took a special interest in conditions of the head and neck and undertook thousands of operations for goitre. He travelled widely, lecturing about his techniques. He published many articles and designed many instruments. His main legacy for OMFS Surgeons was that he observed that when malignant lymph glands were individually removed from the neck, recurrent disease and death were inevitable. He developed the neck dissection in which he removed all the glands 'en bloc' after clamping the carotid artery; this often resulted in a cure. Now, over 100 years later, we routinely carry out a modification of his operation and afterwards sew up with his needle holders.*

[5]*Thomas Ponfret Kilner (1890-1964) was one of the four original plastic surgeons who developed hospital departments, in his case at the Queen Mary Hospital Roehampton, for the treatment of facial injuries sustained in the two world wars (The others were Gillies, McIndoe & Rainsford Mowlem). Kilner consulted at many hospitals around London and wrote about cleft lip and palate deformity and war injuries. He became Professor of Plastic Surgery at Oxford and was twice President of the British Association of Plastic Surgeons. He designed several surgical instruments which bear his name.*

[6]*Sir Archibald McIndoe (1900 - 1960) moved to England from his native New Zealand in 1930 where he joined his cousin Harold Gillies in private practice. After a spell with the American Royal College of Surgeons, he became Consultant Plastic Surgeon to the Royal Air Force just before the Second World War. As war broke out McIndoe moved to the newly rebuilt Queen Victoria Hospital, East Grinstead, subsequently forming the Centre for Plastic and Jaw Injuries. There he treated many burns and facial injuries; he was an innovator and teacher. He was a founding member of the British Association of Plastic Surgeons and later President. He was Knighted in 1947 and became President of the Royal College of Surgeons in 1958.*

[7]*Oscar Huntington Allis (1836 - 1921) practised orthopaedic surgery in Philadelphia. His chief specialism was trauma. He is known for Allis's sign in fractured neck of femur, for his splint, his dissector and his forceps, which were originally designed to retract the peritoneum*

[8]*Bernard Rudolf Konrad von Langenbeck (1810 - 1887)* was a Professor of Surgery in Berlin. He was widely known for his technique of sub-periosteal dissection for cleft palates. He discovered the yeast that we know now as candida albicans.

Instruments used chiefly for bone, orthognathic surgery and trauma

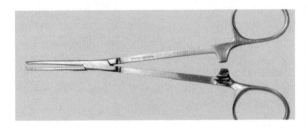

Kocher's[1] forceps. These have interlocking terminal teeth and were designed to be used as arterial clamps. We use them as bone holding forceps.

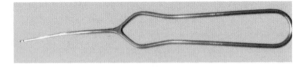

Kelsey Fry[2] bone awl. To pass wires through soft tissues & around bone, usually mandible. The wire is initially fed through the hole near the tip.

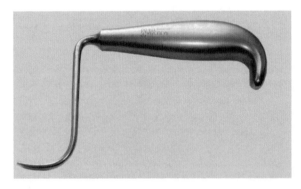

Tessier[3] mobilizer. Used in pairs to pull forward the maxilla which has been divided.

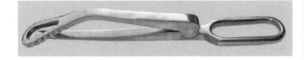

Rowe's[4] Malar elevator. Used to lift a fractured malar from beneath the zygomatic arch. (Gillies's lift)

[1] *Emil Theodor Kocher (1841 - 1917) was a German Professor of Surgery in Berne. He introduced a submandibular approach for removing cancer of the tongue. He developed several surgical instruments and was awarded the Nobel Prize for Surgery in 1911.*

[2] *Sir William Kelsey Fry (1889 - 1963) obtained dental and medical qualifications and worked during the First World War with Gillies at Queen Mary Hospital, Sidcup. Between the world wars he worked at Guy's and during the second war at East Grinstead. Following his retirement from Guy's in 1949 he moved to the Institute of Dental Surgery as Consultant in Oral Surgery and was subsequently Dean of the Faculty of Dental Surgery of the Royal College of Surgeons of England.*

[3] *Paul Tessier (1917 -2008) is regarded as the founder of Cranio-Facial surgery. He developed early interests in cleft lip & palate and Dupuytren's contracture but subsequently became involved with plastic surgery and burns as well as ophthalmology. He used bone grafts to stabilize mid facial osteotomies for severe facial deformities, an innovation which decreased relapse.*

[4] *Norman Lestor Rowe (1915 - 1991) was Consultant OMFS surgeon at St Mary's Roehampton and the Westminster and Eastman Dental Hospitals. He was known affectionately, to his colleagues and trainees, as 'Uncle'. He initially worked in dental practice but during WW II joined the Dental Corps where he became involved in treating facial injuries. Later he undertook medical and surgical training and was appointed as a Consultant at Rooksdown House Basingstoke where he worked with Gillies. After the unit moved to Roehampton he co wrote 'Fractures of the Facial Skeleton' with Killey, published in 1955, and later 'Maxillofacial Injuries', co-written with John Williams and published in 1985. This was, and remains, a defining text on the subject. Rowe was an innovator in the surgery of secondary cleft deformity and temporomandibular joint ankylosis. He trained many aspiring OMFS surgeons and gained wide respect and influence in the management roles he undertook. He was a defining influence on the development of OMFS as practised in the UK today.*

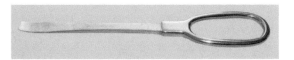

Bristow's malar elevator.   Used for the same purpose. The orthopaedic surgeons use the same instrument as a periosteal elevator, for which it was designed. Walter Rowley Bristow (1882 - 1947)

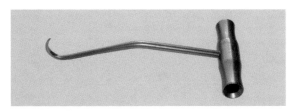

Poswillo's[5] hook. Also used to pull out a fractured malar.

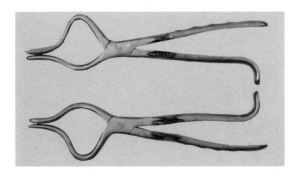

Rowe's dis-impaction forceps. Used in pairs to pull a displaced fractured maxilla forward or to move a divided maxilla forward during orthognathic surgery.

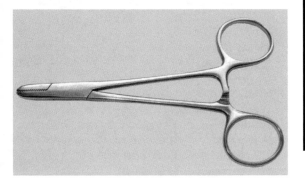

Lawson Tait[6] forceps. Used for tightening wires, they were designed for soft tissues.

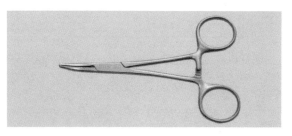

[7]Spencer Wells forceps. Used for feeding wires between teeth they were designed as artery clamps.

[5]*David Poswillo (1927 - 2003) an OMFS surgeon, came to London from New Zealand at the age of 36 to work at the Royal College of Surgeons and subsequently at the Queen Victoria Hospital, East Grinstead. He undertook innovative research in teratology and later became head of Craniofacial Surgery at Adelaide University. He returned to London to be Professor of Oral Surgery at the Royal Dental Hospital and, when that hospital closed, Guy's. He chaired the Department of Health working party on anaesthesia in dentistry, which improved safety, and later the government committee on tobacco and health.*

[6] *Robert Lawson Tait (1845 - 1899) was born and educated in Scotland. He practised gynaecology in Birmingham. He wrote his textbook 'Diseases of Women' in 1877 as well as many other books and papers. He was a controversial figure and, for a time, was the most famous surgeon of his day. He was visited by surgeons from Europe and the USA and travelled to Canada to teach. He was a founding member and President of the British Gynaecology Society.*

[7]*Sir Thomas Spencer Wells (1818 - 1897) was a pioneering gynaecologist at the Samaritan Free Hospital for Women and Children in London. He established ovariotomy, was a champion for public health and a rival of Lawson Tait; he became President of the Royal College of Surgeons.*

31. <u>Minor Oral Surgery</u>

About half of all referrals into an OMFS department will be for patients who require some form of minor surgery, most of which will be dento-alveolar. By far the most will be carried out using local anaesthetic. In addition there will be an enormous number of referrals of oral medicine cases, many of whom will end up having biopsies carried out. The collective name given to these procedures is Minor Oral Surgery (MOS).

The arrangements for these procedures will vary between hospitals. In some they will be performed in the operating theatre suite; some will have a dedicated theatre for minor surgery, and in many more they will be carried out in the outpatient facility, often in a dental chair which is also used for consultations.

When operating in a theatre the surgeon will be assisted by a 'scrub nurse' who will be in charge of the instruments and will hand them to the surgeon. For MOS the surgeon will help himself to instruments from the instrument trolley.

We will now introduce you to an MOS procedure to demonstrate the process. A biopsy of a white patch in the floor of mouth is to be performed by the trainee assisted by a staff nurse, (biopsies are often carried out on a biopsy clinic with the surgeon and just one nurse assisting). For surgical procedures involving dental extractions, which may need a drill, or for laser surgery, the surgeon is assisted by two nurses; one scrubs and assists while the other acts as a 'runner', remaining unsterile and fetching equipment, setting up the drill and suction, or programming the laser, just as in the operating theatre.

We would like to say a special word about identification. When carrying out MOS there will be a large number of patients having very similar surgery. Whenever there is a possibility that something will go wrong eventually it will and someone may get the wrong operation. In surgical terms this would be a 'never event', i.e. an event that should never happen. We have seen a case where a patient had surgery based on the notes of a different patient with a similar sounding name. Fortunately they both needed the same operation, removal of lower left eight. The patient's name, their hospital number, operative procedure and consent form should be displayed on a board in the operating room, be it theatre or outpatient suite, so that

it can be double checked; this is particularly important for dental extractions. We have seen two instances where a half-witted trainee sent a biopsy specimen and a request form labelled for different patients. This caused considerable correspondence, paperwork and hassle, which went on for months for the Consultant in charge. Always check a patient's name, hospital number, address and date of birth before operating. Never have a second set of notes on a surface with the notes of the patient you are dealing with and never label specimen pots or request forms before they are used.

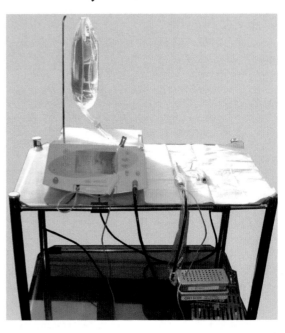

Where surgery requires the use of a drill, suction or laser this will need to be set up before the patient enters the room. A third person should be present to act as 'runner', to fetch and carry things. The drill unit is set up on a trolley with the end of the cord covered with a sterile plastic sheath. Fluid from an IV bag passes to the hand piece through a sterile tube. The drill unit is operated with a foot control which simultaneously pumps the fluid to the bur.

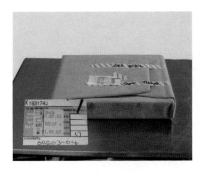

1. Instruments arrive from ASDU (Area Sterilising & Disinfection Unit) or CSSD (Central Sterile Services Department) wrapped in paper and closed with autoclave tape. Each has a label (inset) which identifies the instruments. This is placed in the patient's notes so the instruments can be traced should there be any contamination issue later.

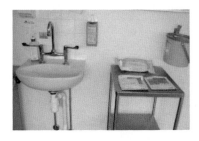

2. The room must have a wash basin with taps that can be elbow operated, surgical scrub, a flat surface for the surgical gown and gloves, and a sharps disposal bin.

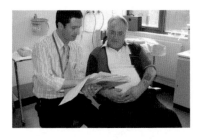

3. The patient is identified by checking their name, address and date of birth against the notes. The patient should already have given informed consent for the procedure.

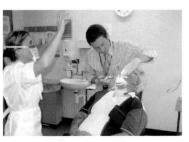

4. Local anaesthetic is administered by the surgeon wearing non sterile examination gloves.

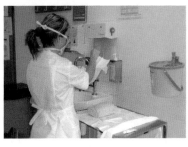

5. Meanwhile the nurse, who is wearing a plastic disposable apron (cheap), scrubs and dons sterile gloves.

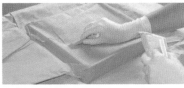

6. The tray of surgical instruments is already on a clean surgical trolley. The outer blue covering has been opened with clean hands from the outside. Now the inner sterile green layer is opened by the nurse wearing sterile gloves.

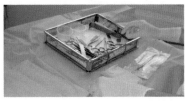

7. The pack contains the instruments and sterile towels to drape the patient.

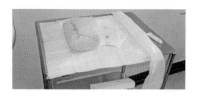

8. The sterile gown for the surgeon has been opened on to a sterile towel with the gloves.

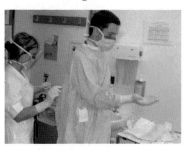

9. The surgeon scrubs, dons gown & gloves, while the nurse ties up from behind. The surgeon's gown is sterile, the ties are behind so may be tied with or without sterile gloves.

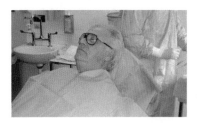

10. The patient is covered by a sterile gown from the tray with another behind his head. He wears protective wide lens safety spectacles.

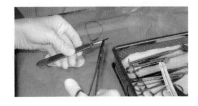

11. The blade is placed on the handle (unless a disposable scalpel is used) and the suture mounted on the needle holder.

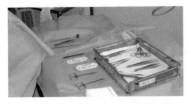

12. Instruments most likely to be used have been laid out of the tray with sutures and swabs.

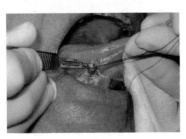

13. The procedure is carried out by the surgeon who helps himself to instruments from the tray and is assisted by the nurse.

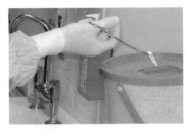

14. When finished, the surgeon disposes of the blade, suture and needle into the sharps bin.

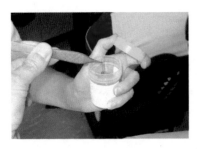

15. The specimen is placed into the specimen pot.

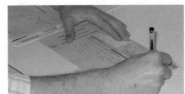

16. The surgeon writes up the operation note and pathology request on a form or electronically using the hospital's clinical records system. Always check that the labels on the specimen pot and request form are for the correct patient.

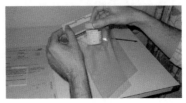

17. The specimen pot is placed into the envelope on the back of the pathology request form and sealed.

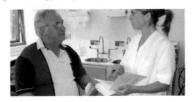

18. The nurse goes through the post-operative instruction leaflet with the patient.

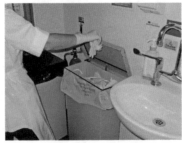

19. Contaminated disposables, like gloves, swabs etc, are placed into a yellow clinical waste bag. Uncontaminated material, such as wrapping paper, are placed in a black household waste bag (cheaper to dispose of).

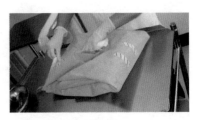

20. The used instruments are wrapped up.

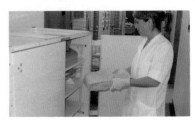

21. The wrapped instruments are placed into the contaminated instruments trolley which is returned to the sterile supply department at the end of the day.

32. <u>The Management of Impacted Teeth</u>

An oral & maxillofacial surgery hospital department should provide you with plenty of opportunity to receive the supervised instruction necessary to become a safe dento-alveolar surgeon. Much of this work comprises of removal of impacted third molars which for historical reasons has been referred into hospitals. We regard this with some regret as nearly all of it could be carried out in general dental practice by general dentists. Although some cases can be technically difficult the skills to do it can be acquired by a competent practitioner in a few weeks of supervised instruction and practice.

Mandibular third molars normally erupt between the ages of 18 and 24 years. Vertically aligned teeth will generally erupt fully but may become impacted in soft tissue if there is insufficient room in the dental arch; this may become the cause of repeated pericoronal infection. Mesially inclined teeth may gradually become vertical after eruption or impact further; they too may lead to pericoronitis, exacerbate oral hygiene and predispose to caries in the distal of the second molar; they may become carious themselves. In any of these cases surgical removal is indicated. There is very little indication for removal of unerupted third molars.

As with all but emergency cases the patients will initially be seen for a consultation in an outpatient clinic and an assessment carried out. Each tooth that is listed for surgery should have the reason recorded in the patients notes and decisions should be made according to the recommendations of the National Institute for Health and Care Excellence (NICE). These are only guidelines so may be varied from in individual cases but the reason must be justifiable and recorded in the patient's records. During the consultation the patient should have the risks and benefits explained to

---

Third Molar Surgery Side Effects Warnings
Pain
Discomfort on eating
Swelling Bleeding
Bruising

Complications Warnings
Infection - pain
Numbness or tingling of lip or tongue with small risk of permanence
Tingling of lip

---

them so that they may give informed consent for the procedure. Normally the patient should be listed for the surgical extractions to be carried out under local anaesthesia; sedation may be used for those who are apprehensive. Many surgeons carry out the surgery under general anaesthesia on a 'day-stay' basis. We think this is wasteful of resources and only rarely indicated.

When assessing the patient consideration should be given to the angulation of the tooth. Mesioangular are the easiest to remove followed by deeper vertical teeth with distoangular impactions the most difficult. Obviously superficially placed teeth are easier to remove than deep. It is unusual for unerupted teeth to need removal as they infrequently lead to pathology.

We mentioned the NICE guidelines for removal of third molars. We will now mention the history of this as it is relevant to current debate within the speciality. In 1997 the Royal College of Surgeons of England published a report and recommendations: 'The Management of Patients with Third Molar (Wisdom) Teeth'. This was soon followed, in 2000 by the National Institute for Health and Care Excellence (NICE) to publish its 'Technology Appraisal Guidance': 'Guidance on the Extraction of Wisdom Teeth'. The NICE document was very welcome because it laid down sensible guidance on when third molars should be removed and recommended no prophylactic surgery where there were no disease and no symptoms; it was a sensible disincentive to unnecessary surgery. However it made no difference to the clinical practice of those of us who already applied sound common sense to our practice. NICE very reasonably intended to review the guidance when the results of two expected controlled clinical trials were published. However these trials did not materialise so there was no review.

More recently it has been suggested that most of the third molar surgery stopped by NICE was needed eventually and was thus carried out on patients at an older age and that they suffered greater side effects and complications as a result. Furthermore non removal of asymptomatic mesioangular impacted teeth predisposed to caries in the second molar which would not occur had the third molar been removed earlier. Clinical guidelines in other countries vary from that of NICE. In 2014 NICE reviewed the issues and decided not to vary its guidance.

In hospital practice the decisions and recommendations to patients will be made by the surgeon and will be based on the best interest of the patient and the culture we come from and work in, without regard to the financial or other considerations; this is one of the key strengths of our National Health Service. Part of this culture is that we do not promote operative treatment, with all its side effects and potential complications, in circumstances where there are no symptoms or disease, unless there is the strongest possible evidence that it will be of benefit to the patient and that not operating might have the severest consequence. We believe that strongest evidence and severest consequence do not presently exist. Whereas we have complete confidence in the probity and unbiased impartiality of NICE we are unsure of the influences bearing on those writing guidance for use in other healthcare systems.

However, where a patient has a part erupted mesioangular impacted third molar and poor oral hygiene with demineralisation of the distal of the second molar, then removal of the third molar should be discussed and possibly recommended to them. When any operation is planned there should be a clear reason (justification) written in the patient's notes and this should be done for each individual third molar. In the case of an upper tooth which may be left unopposed by the removal of a lower this may be sufficient justification as removal should produce minimal side effects and complications.

Two particular complications of third molar removal need consideration as there is some variance in opinion and practice. These are injury to the lingual and inferior alveolar nerves. Lingual nerve damage, although unusual, can be very disturbing for the patient and lead to disabling allodynia which is worse than anaesthesia. Most injuries are temporary in nature and usually result in paraesthesia which gradually recovers over a couple of weeks. This is most frequently caused by the placement of a retractor between the lingual mucoperiosteum and bone; most frequently used is a

NICE indications for third molar removal

Unrestorable caries
Untreatable pulpal or periapical pathology
Cellulitis, abscess, osteomyelitis
Resorption of the tooth or adjacent teeth
Fracture of tooth
Cyst or tumour of the follicle
Tooth impeding surgery e.g. tumour resection or reconstruction

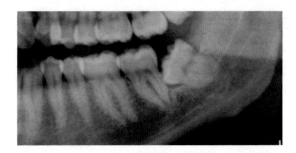

The tooth is inclined mesially and has been causing recurrent pericoronitis. The roots are close to the ID canal. Mesio-angular teeth are usually easier to remove than disto-angular or even many vertical teeth.

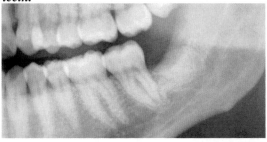

A coronectomy has been carried out on this tooth with the root close to the ID canal. Coronectomy makes the surgery easier and quicker for the patient. The remaining root often migrates upwards but needs subsequent removal infrequently. Sometimes the procedure fails when a conical root comes out completely when not intended. It should not be done for severely carious or non vital teeth.

Haworth's retractor. If this instrument is used to protect the nerve from a rotating bur it will be inadequate. A surgeon who removes lingual bone before elevating the tooth should not rely only on this retractor. Alternatively buccal bone can be removed and the tooth split to avoid the necessity to remove disto-lingual bone.

However, there can be no doubt that many surgeons have removed third molars for years without causing damage to the nerve and have relied on their knowledge of the anatomy to avoid the nerve completely; if this technique is to be used then the placement of a lingual retractor, so that the area of operation can be adequately visualised, is desirable. Many of the nerve injuries have been caused simply by placement of a retractor. This is principally due to inexperienced surgeons attempting to lift a flap too far forward; it is easier to lift the periosteum from the bone starting in the region of the bottom of the ascending ramus of the mandible. Cutting the tooth up from an

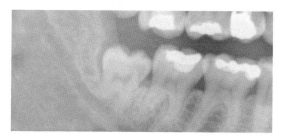

Here the distal root is dilacerated (bent) by it's close relationship to the ID canal. If the tooth is asymptomatic and there is no caries it can be retained. If there is pericoronitis or caries in the 7 or 8 it can be removed by splitting it vertically and removing the roots separately or a coronectomy carried out.

entirely buccal approach will avoid the problem but will take longer in many cases and of course is more uncomfortable for the patient.

The worse scenario is that if the bur injures the nerve directly, the surgeon is unlikely to know this has happened until it is realised that sensation has not recovered several weeks after surgery. In this case the severed nerve will have retracted. If sensation is still abnormal the nerve may be surgically explored, scar tissue removed and an attempt made to suture the ends of the damaged nerve together. Results from this are disappointing but may be better than nothing; an attempt should be considered if the nerve has not recovered after 3 months.

Third molar roots may on occasion be intimately related to the inferior dental nerve and cause compression of the nerve during surgery. A close relationship of the tooth roots to the nerve can usually be predicted from a digital orthopantomographic X-ray image. Where there is doubt a more accurate image may be made with a cone beam computerised tomograph (CT) scan which will demonstrate the relationship of the roots to the inferior dental bundle. However, although a CT scan will give a better image of the relationship to the inferior dental bundle to the

X-ray signs of close root and ID bundle relation
Interruption of white lines of ID canal
Lucency across third molar root
Deviation of the canal
Narrowing of tooth root
Deflection of tooth root by canal
A better image is obtained by a CT scan but an improved outcome for the patient is yet to be proved

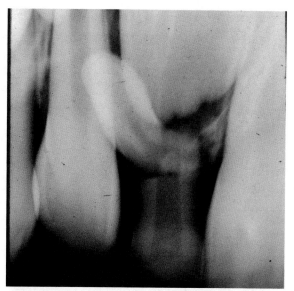

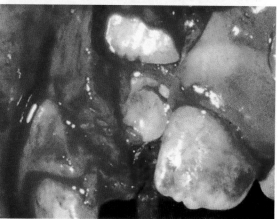

A supernumerary tooth is preventing the eruption of this permanent central incisor as seen on X-ray (top) and at operation below. Surgical removal of the supernumerary will allow the incisor to erupt. There is a lot of this minor work.

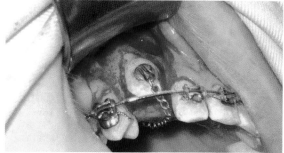

An unerupted canine has been exposed and an orthodontic bracket and chain attached with light cured acid etch seen here before wound closure

Complication

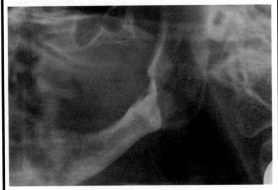

An unerupted third molar has become exposed to the mouth consequent upon alveolar bone resorption. Now causing discomfort beneath a denture and carious it needs removing.

The weakened mandible has now fractured as a result of the surgery.

Nomenclature

Anaesthesia:- absence of sensation

Hypoaesthesia:- diminished sensation

Paraesthesia:- abnormal sensation

Dyaesthesia:- unpleasant sensation

Hyperalgesia:- increased response to a normally painful stimulus

Allodynia:- pain response to stimulus not normally painful

tooth roots, it has not been proved that this translates into less permanent nerve damage. In order to justify the additional radiation, expense and inconvenience of this, or indeed any, investigation it should be proved that it may influence a change in the management of the patient. Injury to the inferior alveolar nerve can be avoided by splitting the tooth vertically for removal or simply leaving part of the root in place during surgery (coronectomy), a technique which not only has few complications but is easily accomplished and may be less uncomfortable for the patient than removing the whole of a root with unfavourable morphology. Damage to the inferior dental nerve does not require exploratory surgery unless it is obvious a root fragment has been pushed into the canal. Paraesthesia is usually, but not always, temporary and allodynia is very rare. Indeed iatrogenic injury to the inferior dental nerve occurs very frequently during orthognathic surgery as it is impossible to split the mandible sagittally without some trauma to it. Some permanent disturbance of sensation of the skin of the chin regularly occurs without causing disability.

A frequent request from orthodontists is for surgical help with ectopic maxillary canines. Infrequently this is to request their removal if they are very ectopic and their position and the age of the patients suggests that they may cause resorption of the permanent incisors. More frequently we are asked to surgically uncover them to facilitate their eruption or traction into the dental arch.

Much has been written about the diagnosis of their exact position with two x-rays using the parallax technique, which students learn about for their examinations, or cone beam CT scans. Usually this is not necessary as often the tooth can be seen or palpated buccal of the dental or in the palate. If it cannot be seen or palpated then it is usually palatal but might be high within the line of the arch. Occasionally the apex of the tooth may be palpated in a high position buccally while the crown is palatal. In these circumstances the surgeon may feel more confident if the precise position has been previously revealed by a cone beam CT scan. Similarly when an unerupted canine is suspected of causing resorption of a maxillary incisor a cone-beam CT scan will reveal the exact position.

Surgery can involve uncovering the tooth and suturing in a temporary pack to form a channel for eruption, the open technique. Alternatively the tooth may be exposed and an orthodontic bracket and chain can be attached to pull the tooth in position, the closed technique. Which is used is the decision of the orthodontist who requests the treatment.

33. <u>Histopathology</u>

All surgeons depend heavily on the services of a histopathology department. Nearly all of the material removed from patients is sent for examination for diagnosis, confirmation of a known or suspected diagnosis, or to check the surgical margins following cancer excision. You will be involved with a pathologist almost from day one; you will be taking biopsies of soft tissue lesions from within the mouth and will inevitably be asked to fill in request forms and label specimen bottles. You should attempt to get to know your friendly pathologist; he or she will almost certainly be keen to discuss specimens with you. Hopefully there will be clinico-pathological conferences (CPCs) in your department where you can discuss clinical cases and look at the histopathology slides together. An understanding of pathology is essential to understanding disease; it will enrich your clinical learning and help with your postgraduate examinations.

You will inevitably be called upon to remove a number of benign lesions from the mouth. These are all sent for histology to check the diagnosis, for, although we are certain of a benign (not cancerous) diagnosis, occasionally we may be wrong and furthermore the patient and their GP also need to be reassured. When a lesion is removed entirely and sent for examination the procedure is called an 'excisional biopsy' as opposed to an 'incisional biopsy' where a part of the lesion is removed. You should say on the request form which it is.

You should make your requests for histopathology with a clear, but not verbose, clinical history. In many hospitals these requests will be made on the Trust's computer system via their Care Records System (CRS). Where they are still made on handwritten request forms it will be appreciated if they are written legibly. You should include reference to any previous specimens and their laboratory numbers. Always make sure you have correctly labelled both the request form and the specimen bottle. For some oral lesions, such as suspected lichen planus, the history should include current drugs taken. For white patches the pathologist should be told about smoking and drinking habits. We also encourage you to put down a short list of differential diagnoses.

The pathology report will include a macroscopic description of the specimen, a microscopic description

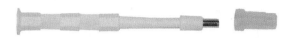

Disposable punch used for taking small biopsies. This is most useful for attached gingiva and for taking multiple samples from extensive white patches

of the material and a conclusion on the diagnosis; for a cancer resection a comment will be made on the clearance at the margins of the lesion.

The pathological diagnosis may not be taken as gospel truth in every case. Sometimes a poor specimen has been provided, particularly one too small. Sometimes the specimen may be unrepresentative of the whole lesion. Remember that part of a white patch may show no dysplasia at all whereas a few millimetres away a small invasive cancer may be developing. What is described as mildly, moderately or severely dysplastic will depend upon the individual pathologist's judgement and all of us are fallible. Therefore clinical decisions on management should not be based exclusively on the histology report, although it will be very strong evidence. If a malignancy is suspected on clinical grounds but the histology fails to find any the patient must not be dismissed but followed up and re-biopsy carried out if the lesion does not resolve quickly. Some pathological appearances, especially of bone, may represent a spectrum of abnormal activity such as fibrous dysplasia, ossifying fibroma and osteogenic sarcoma. Here the pathologist may wish to see the X-rays or get the opinion of others. The bone tumour panel consists of a network of pathologists with a special interest in bony lesions; they will pass around borderline or other difficult specimens by post to provide supplementary opinions and reports.

In some cancer cases specimens will be taken after the tumour has been resected to check that the margins have been cleared. The specimens will go straight to the laboratory where they will be frozen and stained before being examined by the pathologist who will give a verbal report to the surgeon in the operating theatre by telephone. This process is known as taking 'frozen sections'.

The Laboratory Process

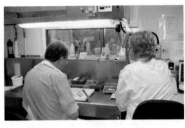
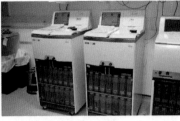
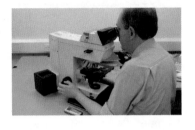

1. The process starts in the 'cut up' room. The pathologist is assisted by a secretary to whom he dictates his findings and measurements.

5. The machines remove all the moisture from the samples using various solvents.

8. The processed slides are presented to the pathologist who looks at them under the microscope and dictates his report. After typing by the secretary, a hard copy goes back to the pathologist who checks there are no mistakes; he then signs to 'authorise' it.

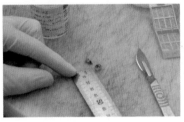

2. The specimen is described and measured for the macroscopic part of the report.

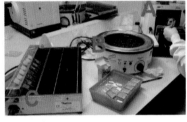

6. Slides are made from the wax blocks. The wax block is frozen, which facilitates easier cutting, and then sliced into thin layers with the microtome (A). A spatula is then used to transfer the wax sections into the water bath (B) where they float. A glass slide is then passed beneath the floating specimen and it is caught onto the slide which is then dried (C).

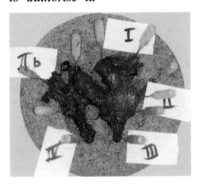

Block dissection of lymph glands from the neck of a patient with intra oral carcinoma. The oncology team will want to know if any of the 40 plus glands in the specimen contain any cancer cells and if so whether there is any spread outside the capsule of the gland. This information is needed to stage the tumour and decide if post-operative radiotherapy is needed. The specimen has been pegged onto a cork board by the surgeon to help the pathologist orientate it and work out at what level in the neck he is taking glands from. A neck dissection will be time consuming work for the histopathologist. The levels of the neck 1, 2, 2b, 3 & 4 have been marked.

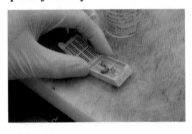

3. Pieces of the specimen are cut off and placed in a labelled cassette for processing into wax.

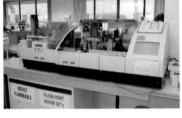

7. The slides then pass through the staining machine; this one is staining with haematoxylin and eosin.

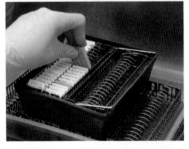

4. The cassette is placed, with others, in the rack for processing.

34. <u>Venepuncture - Taking a Blood Sample</u>

Two of the tasks you may be called upon to perform are to bleed patients for haematological, biochemical or immunological testing or to place intravenous cannulae to be used to deliver parenteral fluids or medication.

The need for you to bleed patients will depend upon the availability of phlebotomists. In some hospitals they carry out this task not only for outpatients who need investigations but do a round of the wards each morning. To avail yourself of this service you will need to make an on-line request or write a request card the night before or early in the morning before they arrive. Similarly intravenous catheters may be placed by clinical support workers but this may not be the case in many establishments so if there are none, or they are not around, the task will fall on you.

Venepuncture will be a useful skill to learn if you are ever going to work in a situation where you will be giving intravenous sedation. Your hospital appointment will give you ample opportunity to learn and become practised.

Before you start you should prepare yourself by learning what equipment you need, how to use it and how to select suitable veins. You should be organised and practise on a manikin before starting on patients. The operating theatre is an ideal place to get practice as the anaesthetist will be putting an IV cannula into every patient who is having an anaesthetic and most will be happy to teach and supervise you.

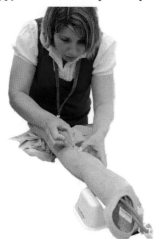

Practise on a manikin before starting on patients.

The Closed Vacuum system

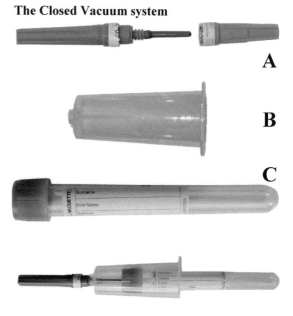

Here is a 21 gauge needle with a valve (A), a hollow plastic tube that the needle screws onto (B), and a vacuumed blood sample bottle (C). This has a rubber bung on the end which is inserted into the tube after the needle has been inserted into the vein. Blood flows into the tube, encouraged by the vacuum. The vacuum is such that flow stops when there is sufficient blood. The valve allows the bottle to be removed while the needle is still in the vein without spillage so that another tube can be attached for a different test.

There are several commercially available closed systems for taking blood. They have several advantages over using a hypodermic syringe and needle. The main one is that the blood goes straight into the collecting bottle without the need to decant it, leading to less risk of spillage and injury from the needle.

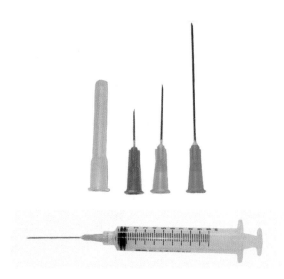

First choose a vein that can be seen and can be felt. If there are none your second choice is one that can be felt but not seen. A vein that can be seen but not felt should be your last choice but it will be difficult. An elderly person may have veins that can be easily felt but are nevertheless difficult to cannulate and withdraw blood.

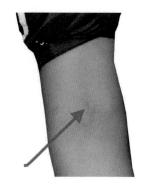

Hypodermic needles and syringe for venepuncture

All equipment for intravenous access is colour coded. A green needle (21 gauge) is the smallest that can be used to take blood samples. A smaller needle will cause the blood to haemolyse (damage to the cell walls leading to release of their contents into the plasma). This will give inaccurate results, particularly for haemoglobin or potassium.

A hypodermic needle and syringe may still be the easiest way of bleeding a patient if they have small or otherwise difficult veins, such as might be the case if they have been damaged by a drug abuse habit.

When using a syringe to take blood you should be careful to withdraw the plunger only very gently and not squirt the blood out quickly through the needle which will also cause haemolysis. The smaller needles (blue 23 gauge and orange 25 gauge) should only be used for injecting medication; they are too small for taking blood. The larger the gauge number the smaller is the outside diameter of the needle.

Choosing a vein

When finding a vein to take blood from, the arm should be compressed by a tourniquet, a blood pressure cuff or by an assistant. The pressure applied should be between systolic and diastolic blood pressure so that arterial blood will flow into the arm but venous flow out is occluded. The vein will be encouraged to stand out if it is warm, if the hand is repeatedly made into a fist to pump the blood and if the vein is tapped gently with your hand.

The ante-cubital fossa is the best site for taking blood from adults.

Ask the patient to repeatedly make a fist which encourages blood flow so that the vein stands out more.

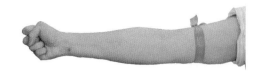

Tapping the vein with your finger will also encourage it to be prominent.

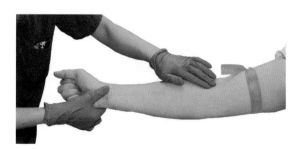

Equipment needed for taking blood

Trolley
Sharps bin
A high sided tray for equipment
A paper towel or pad to absorb any spilt blood
PPE (gloves and apron) x 2

Hand sanitizer
Chlorhexidine wipes for trolley and tray
Disposable tourniquet
Chlorhexidine wipe for skin
Blood bottles and request form as appropriate
Cotton wool swab and tape to secure it to skin

Venepuncture Preparation (away from patient)

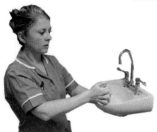

1. Decontaminate Hands

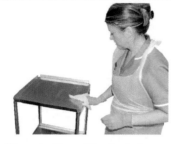

3. Clean trolley with alcohol wipe

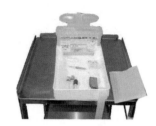

5. Equipment collected in tray on trolley ready to take to patient

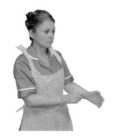

2. Put on PPE

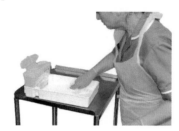

4. Clean inside of tray

Venepuncture procedure

Approach the patient with a cool confident air and appear calm even though you may not be. Taking blood from a conscious patient for the first few times is the best opportunity for a new house surgeon to demonstrate his or her inexperience and make a fool of themselves. It is worse than giving your first ID block as the patient will be able to see every move you make.

Then follow this procedure;

1. Introduce yourself

2. Identify patient by name, date of birth and hospital number

3. On the patient check any in-patient identity band against hospital records.

4. Explain what you intend to do and why.

5. Explain side-effects (bruising bleeding discomfort etc).

6. Ask about any medical history possible complications e.g. bleeding problem, latex allergy.

7. Ask if they have has samples taken before, enquire about any preferred veins for sampling.

8. Make patient comfortable supporting arm.

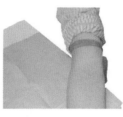

9. Apply tourniquet and identify vein.

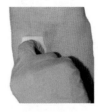

10. Clean the skin over the vein with a disposable alcohol wipe.

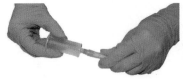

11. Screw the needle onto the hub.

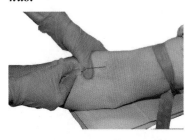

12. Apply traction to skin below and to side of vein to immobilize the vein.

13. Advance needle through skin and into vein bevel up at about 30 degrees.

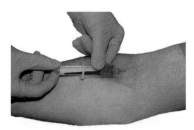

14. Release traction when needle is in the vein, push the vacuumed specimen tube into the hub so that it engages with the needle valve; the required amount of blood will flow into the bottle.

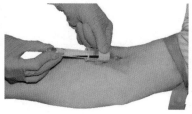

15. If you need another sample for a different test remove the bottle and replace it with another.

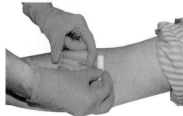

16. Remove the last bottle, release the tourniquet then remove the needle while applying pressure with cotton wool, tape the cotton wool down.

17. Place the needle in the sharps box and clean up the equipment, remove gloves and de-contaminate hands.

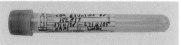

18. Fill in request form and label the bottle or make request on-line through patient records system as appropriate for your hospital. If your hospital used electronic requests you may have to print a bar code to stick on the specimen bottle. Always print patient's full name on requests and bottles. Document in patients notes. Place specimens in transport bag to go to laboratory

Failure

If, after two attempts, you have failed to get blood from the patient you should withdraw from the field of battle and retire to regroup. If the patient is in pain, passed out, or worse still taking the piss, if he is covered with blood or there is a pile of blood stained swabs or blood in the bed sheets then it is time to give up and ask someone else to do it.

However, if you have maintained your dignity without causing a mess then blame the patient's awkward veins and consider your options. Tidy up, throw away the used sharps and swabs and, if you consider you have a reasonable chance of success, permit yourself one (but only one) further attempt before asking someone else to do it.

35. <u>Venepuncture - Inserting a Venflon IV Cannula</u>

<u>The Venflon winged intravenous cannula</u>

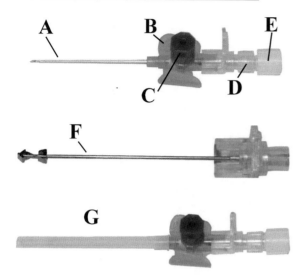

Colour	Gauge size	Used for
Blue	22G	Crystalloid
Pink	20G	Crystalloid & Colloid
Green	18G	Crystalloid, colloid & blood
Grey	16G	Crystalloid, colloid & blood
Orange	14G	Crystalloid, colloid & blood

The venflon consists of a plastic cannula (A), with wings, (B), to facilitate attachment to the skin. There is a side port (C) for attachment of a syringe to administer intravenous medication. The cannula has a port at the end (D) which can be capped (E) or used to attach an intravenous giving set. The catheter is mounted on a needle (F) which protrudes from the end of the plastic cannula for Venepuncture. When the needle is removed from the plastic cannula a safety device attached to the sharp end is activated. The assembled venflon (G) comes mounted within a protective plastic sheath.

<u>Colour Coding for Cannulae</u>

Cannulae are coding according to gauge size. The larger the size of the catheter the more easily fluid can pass through it. The minimum size for giving fluids would be a 22 gauge (colour coded blue). The minimum size for giving blood products would be an 18 (colour green). A larger gauge 16 (coloured grey) is more reliable & a 14 (coloured orange) would be best. The most commonly used sizes in adults are 20 (pink) and 18 (green).

<u>Choosing a vein</u>

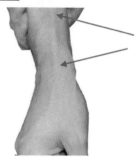

Veins on the lateral side of the wrist are very suitable for IV drips (use the non-dependent arm). It can be painful but a small bleb of local anaesthetic (without vasoconstrictor) adjacent to the vein will be helpful.

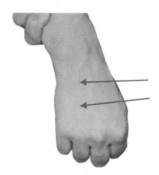

However, the back of the hand is used more often for cannulae used for medication.

Equipment needed for cannulation

Cannula pack (see illustration) and correct size cannula
Disposable tourniquet
Sharps bin
Tray
5 to 10 mls of 0.9% saline flush
smallest cannula needed for the task (giving IV fluids or medication).

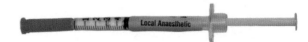

In addition you may like to use some 2% plain lignocaine (not with vasoconstrictor) drawn into a syringe with a small gauge needle. This may be placed into the skin adjacent to the vein to make the process more comfortable for the patient.

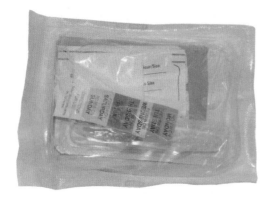

Cannulation Pack

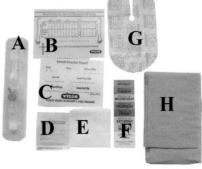

Typical contents of IV Cannulation Pack:-

A: venflon bivalve cannula B: VIP score card (Visual Infusion Phlebitis: a score of 2 indicates the cannula should be replaced i.e. 2 of pain, swelling or erythema.) C: placement record label D: alcohol wipe E: sterile swabs F: day review labels G: dressing H: sterile drape

----

Venepuncture Procedure

1. Clean hands, put on gloves, place sterile towel beneath patient's hand to create a sterile field.

2. Introduce yourself, identify patient, explain and get verbal consent as for venepuncture

3. Position patient comforta.ble

4. Find suitable vein.

5. Apply tourniquet 10 cms above.

6. Palpate straight rebounding vein.

7. Release tourniquet.

8. Open cannula pack onto the tray.

9. Ensure clinical waste bin or bag is available.

10. Activate the flush.

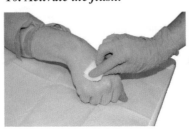

11. Clean skin with alcohol or chlorhexidine wipe for 30 seconds and allow to dry.

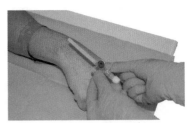

12. Straighten the cannula wings.

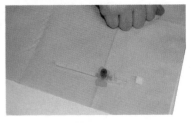

13. Remove the bung and place along with cannula on sterile towel.

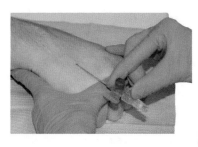

14. Remove the needle cover from the cannula, stabilize the vein by stretching the skin over the vessel with your thumb. Insert the needle through the skin and into the vein with the bevel up at an angle of 15 to 30 degrees.

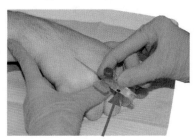

15. As soon as the first flash back is seen lower the cannula so that it is parallel to the arm. Advance further 1 to 2 mms.

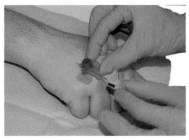

16. Withdraw the needle 2 to 3 mms and observe a second flashback long the length of the cannula. Release the tourniquet and advance the cannula fully into the vein.

17. Apply pressure to the vein above the insertion site with your forefinger.

18. Secure the cannula with your thumb and remove and dispose of the needle into the sharps bin.

19. Attach the white bung to the cannula.

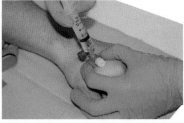

20. Flush with 5 mls saline and ask patient to report any discomfort and observe for any resistance, these would indicate that the cannula is misplaced. Dispose of the flush.

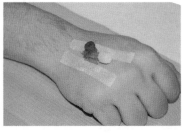

21. Secure the cannula using 2 sterile strips.

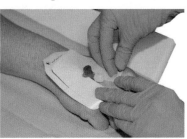

22. Apply dressing.

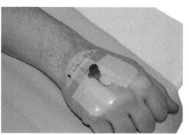

23. Apply label to dressing with initials of person siting the cannula and date and time of insertion.

24. Dispose of gloves and apron.

25. Clean hands.

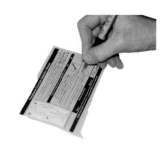

26. Fill in IV form and apply cannula produce sticker if available, record the date time site and name and status of person siting the cannula.

27. Document in patient's notes.

36. <u>Blood Tests: Ordering and Interpretation</u>

Blood tests are an essential tool for us in the management of patients treated in OMFS. Tests carried out in the haematology and biochemistry laboratories (recently combined and renamed Blood Sciences) can seem complicated but are much simpler when viewed from the perspective of the limited number of tests we use and the circumstances in which they may be useful. We will discuss the tests we commonly use, the basis for them and how they may help us.

The request form should be completed legibly and with care. In many hospitals requests must be made on-line; in this case the patient will be given a printed request for the phlebotomist with a bar code for exact identification. Outpatients and inpatients whose blood tests can be anticipated may be bled by a phlebotomist but you may have to do it yourself for urgent unplanned ward admissions if there is no clinical support worker available to do it. Request forms, if used, may be labelled with a sticky label from the patient's notes but blood specimen bottles should be identified with the patient's details in handwriting to reduce the risk of identity error. When requesting blood for transfusion both form and blood specimen bottle must be hand written.

The results will need to be interpreted intelligently and matched to the clinical problem being considered. Usually a reference range will accompany the result which does not necessarily equate with 'normal' in every case. The individual result may be affected by the patient's age, sex, ethnicity, medication, alcohol taken or the time of day; they may also be affected by pregnancy. The result obtained should be compared to the reference range which relates to the range of results for a normal population; this will therefore depend upon the population being compared. 2.5% of the normal population is removed from the top and bottom ends of the reference range so that a result just outside the range does not necessarily mean the patient is abnormal. 5% of the normal population will have a result outside the reference range or 1:20. Thus the result must be carefully considered with the patient's clinical condition and the results of other investigations.

All results should be followed up; it is unacceptable to request any investigation without looking at the results. For routine investigations the results should be available on the hospital computer system the same day; others may take longer. Sometimes this will be

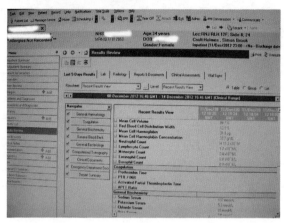

You may have to order tests on a paper request form (as below) or more likely on an on-line clinical records system such as here.

followed by a printed report which should be signed to show it has been looked at and filed in the patient's notes or there may be just an electronic report on the clinical records system which is available for printing if desired. Where a result is outside the reference range a haematologist or biochemist may look at it and make suggestions for further action or investigation.

You should only order tests which are essential for the patient's management. Not only will this avoid incurring the expense of unnecessary tests but it will avoid the problem of trying to interpret the results that are outside the reference range, 5% of which may not represent an abnormality.

All investigations, including blood tests, should be subjected to the "so what" test before they are ordered. This means that you should be clear that the result will have some impact on the management of the patient before you tick the box on the request form or computer screen. You should be clear of the significance of a positive or negative result. Too many investigations are ordered by junior doctors without sufficient justification.

A summary of which blood tests we are likely to use

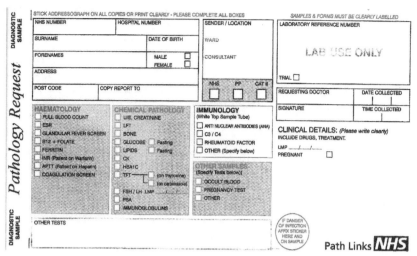

Commonly

Full blood count
• As a baseline measurement of haemoglobin in major cases where significant blood loss is expected.

• Where a patient has bled more than anticipated to check platelets.

• Occasionally if a patient has been anaemic in the past and is due for surgery under anaesthetic.

• Occasionally for a patient with stomatitis (see B12 etc. below).

INR
• Before surgery in a patient taking warfarin but check their anti-coagulant card before testing.

Coagulation screen
• Where there has been inappropriate bleeding.

Urea/Electrolytes
• Diabetics and patients on diuretics before surgery under anaesthetic.

• Rarely in patients with renal disease who are due for surgery.

Glucose
• Diabetics due for surgery under anaesthetic.

• Patients who present with severe infections or unexplained candidiasis.

Sometimes

B12, folate ferritin
• Patients with stomatitis; however, rarely abnormal and of dubious significance.

LFTs
• Patients who present with mouth cancer to check for compromised function which might be caused by metastatic disease or alcohol.

• To check for serum protein levels which might be decreased if nutrition has been compromised by difficulty with eating or high alcohol consumption.

• Patients who present with inappropriate bleeding whose liver dependent clotting factors may be reduced by alcohol or other liver disease.

Occasionally

Anti nuclear antibodies and Rheumatoid factor
• If Sjögren's syndrome is suspected.

Rarely

C4
• As a screening test for hereditary angio-oedema.

Bone and parathyroid hormone
• Where a central giant cell granuloma is found in the jaw to exclude hyper-parathyroidism.

37. <u>Blood Tests - Haematology</u>

Full Blood Count (FBC)

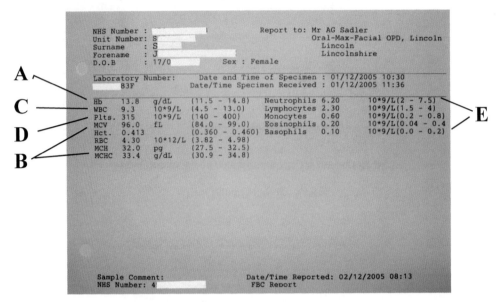

A

C

D

B

E

```
NHS Number :                    Report to: Mr AG Sadler
Unit Number: S                            Oral-Max-Facial OPD, Lincoln
Surname    : S                            Lincoln
Forename   : J                            Lincolnshire
D.O.B      : 17/0         Sex : Female

Laboratory Number:      Date and Time of Specimen : 01/12/2005 10:30
          83F           Date/Time Specimen Received : 01/12/2005 11:36

Hb     13.8   g/dL     (11.5 - 14.8)  Neutrophils 6.20   10*9/L(2 - 7.5)
WBC    9.3    10*9/L   (4.5 - 13.0)   Lymphocytes 2.30   10*9/L(1.5 - 4)
Plts.  315    10*9/L   (140 - 400)    Monocytes   0.60   10*9/L(0.2 - 0.8)
MCV    96.0   fL       (84.0 - 99.0)  Eosinophils 0.20   10*9/L(0.04 - 0.4
Hct.   0.413           (0.360 - 0.460) Basophils  0.10   10*9/L(0.0 - 0.2)
RBC    4.30   10*12/L  (3.82 - 4.98)
MCH    32.0   pg       (27.5 - 32.5)
MCHC   33.4   g/dL     (30.9 - 34.8)



Sample Comment:                 Date/Time Reported: 02/12/2005 08:13
NHS Number: 4                   FBC Report
```

The most frequently used Haematology test in OMFS is the full blood count. This tells us the haemoglobin level and the quantity and proportions of the cellular component of the blood.

A. The most usual need for a full blood count (FBC) is to estimate haemoglobin, most usually as part of pre-operative assessment for anaemia or for a base line assessment to compare with intra-operative measurements in a patient who we expect to lose a significant amount of blood. A low haemoglobin will compromise the oxygen carrying capacity of the blood, which may be important in anaesthesia and surgery for older patients. Any patient with pre-existing cardiac or respiratory disease will be more sensitive to low oxygen availability. An individual can adapt to a low haemoglobin which has been present for some time, for example if they have 'anaemia of chronic disease', especially so if they are fairly inactive. There is therefore no absolute lower haemoglobin level at which a patient can have an anaesthetic. However, a patient who has a low haemoglobin level consequent upon recent blood loss will be much more sensitive and may have a low tolerance to exertion or even be breathless at rest. Therefore patients who have suffered recent trauma and lost blood are more likely to benefit from having a full blood count. In practice we request it pre-operatively for only a few of our patients but we

always would for those undergoing major surgery where a significant amount of blood may be lost, such as resection of oral cancer, orthognathic surgery or a major facial injury. The National Institute of Heath & Care (NICE) has published guidelines as to which patients we should request pre-operative investigations for; this guidance looks as if it has been written by a committee and is over complicated but it is potentially useful in preventing a lot of unnecessary tests.

Occasionally we may request an FBC (together with haematinics) if we see a patient with atrophic glossitis which may be a symptom of chronic iron deficiency anaemia and there is thought to be an association with angular chelitis. Our experience is that requesting an FBC for patients with sore tongues or angular chelitis produces an enormous number of normal results from the laboratory.

B. The red cell indices Mean Cell Volume (MCV), Haematocrit (Ht), Red Blood Cell Concentration (RBCC), Mean Cell Haemoglobin Concentration (MCHC) should be interpreted together. Some are not measured but are mathematically derived from the others. They can, when considered with the clinical picture, give an indication of the possible cause of anaemia. Anaemia with reduced MCV, MCH and MCHC is called hypochromic-microcytic. Iron deficiency anaemia and thalassaemia produce this blood picture as sometimes can 'anaemia of chronic disease'. A normal MCV and MCHC is called normocytic and normochromic anaemia. This will include most anaemias of chronic disease as well as anaemia resulting from blood loss, haemolysis and decreased RBC formation as a consequence of renal failure, aplastic and malignant disease of the marrow. A raised MCV is called macrocytic and mostly results from vitamin B12 and folate deficiency.

If the indices are abnormal the haematologist will examine cells under a microscope as their shape and staining characteristics may help in diagnosis; this will be in the report. Anisocytosis means the red cells vary in size, Poikilocytosis, in shape. The other terms used, macro, micro and normo, you are familiar with.

An increase in the concentration of red cells may be caused by the rare condition polycythaemia ruba vera where there is over activity of the marrow, but it is more commonly caused as an adaption to chronic hypoxia related to lung disease and chronic smoking. A macrocytosis is often caused by excessive alcohol intake.

If haemoglobin and red cells are present in their normal absolute quantities they may still be shown to be in reduced concentration if there is an increase in the volume of the blood plasma; this may occur if a patient has been over-hydrated by intravenous fluids. Similarly, pregnancy increases plasma volume and therefore lower estimations for Hb. and RBC. If a patient is dehydrated then a corresponding increase in concentrations may be recorded.

C. The total white cell count is commonly increased in infection, inflammation or tissue damage. You can expect it to be increased if a patient has a large abscess, particularly if they are systemically unwell with pyrexia, after facial trauma or after major surgery. The count will return to normal as the patient recovers; occasionally serial white counts may be used to monitor recovery but this is unusual in our clinical practice as we can observe recovery directly. The white count may also increase in any malignant disease particularly of the bone marrow (leukaemia).

A decrease in white cells is uncommon but can occur in viral infections and when a patient is overwhelmed by acute sepsis or cancer. It can also occur as a result of chemotherapy. Very low levels will lead to infection from otherwise harmless bacteria and mucosal ulceration may occur. Candidiasis of the mouth is particularly associated with a low WBC.

D. Platelets, which are an essential part of haemostasis, may be decreased in numbers in aplastic anaemia, leukaemia and as a result of chemotherapy or radiotherapy. However, the most common cause of low platelets is autoimmune increased breakdown seen in idiopathic thrombocytopenia purpura (ITP). This may occur as a primary disease, mostly in women, or secondary to other disease processed or caused by some drugs. Most usually we will see patients with low platelets when they need dental extractions, usually because they have ITP or have recently had chemotherapy. However, platelet levels quickly recover after chemotherapy and fluctuate with ITP so the levels should be checked just beforehand. The level needs to be very low before there is a bleeding problem usually below about $60 \times 10^9/L$.

E. The differential white cell count shows the number of the individual types of white cells in the blood. This is of infrequent use to us in OMFS. However we will briefly explain their significance. Neutrophils are the most numerous. They offer protection against bacteria and engage in phagocytosis. They are increased in acute infections, inflammation, tissue damage, where there are solid tumours and chronic myeloid leukaemia. The lymphocytes consist of 70% T – lymphocytes which destroy infected cells and 30% B – lymphocytes which produce antibodies. There are also a few 'Natural Killer' cells. Lymphocytes increase in infectious mononucleosis, several other viral infections, chronic bacterial infections and several rarer diseases which include toxoplasmosis which can present with enlarged lymph nodes in the neck. They are increased in chronic lymphatic leukaemia and non-Hodgkin's lymphoma. Monocytes phagocytose foreign material and have a role in presenting antigens to T lymphocytes; they are rarely increased in number. Eosinophils phagocytose larger foreign material and have a role in killing organisms larger than bacteria. They are present at the site of inflammation caused by allergic reactions such as allergic asthma and hay fever. They are increased in parasitic worm infections and allergic diseases as well as occasionally in Hodgkin's lymphoma. Basophils are rarely seen in the peripheral blood. They become Mast cells in the tissues which release mediators of acute inflammation; they are raised in chronic myeloid leukaemia but rarely otherwise.

Coagulation Studies

Intermittently patients with a history of prolonged or excessive bleeding present needing surgery or dental extraction. The most important part of the investigation is the clinical history but you will need to arrange a full blood count to check their platelet count and a coagulation screen.

The coagulation screen consists of three tests. The prothrombin time (PT) tests the extrinsic coagulation pathway clotting factors and the final common pathway as it forms fibrin. The activated partial thromboplastin time (APTT) assesses the intrinsic and final common pathways and the thrombin time (TT) the final pathway only. If all of these are normal then the coagulation cascade should be normal and produce normal fibrin for haemostasis. If any are abnormal the report will advise what to do next; to retest, do additional investigations or to refer the patient to a haematologist. If the patient is still bleeding a haematologist's help will be needed immediately.

The most common inherited clotting defects are Haemophilia A, followed by Haemophilia B or Christmas Disease. These are caused by deficiency of factors 8 and 9 respectively. They are part of the intrinsic pathway so that the APTT will be prolonged, whereas PT and TT will be normal. More commonly, clotting factors are deficient due to liver disease, which is acquired. PT will be most sensitive to this but in

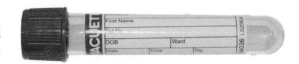

Blood for a full blood count is collected in a lavender topped colour coded bottle. It contains ethylene diamine tetra acetic acid (EDTA) which stops the sample from clotting by removing calcium ions from the plasma.

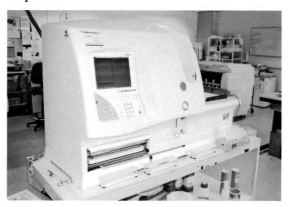

In the laboratory the full blood count is determined by one of these machines. The sample is shaken to ensure even distribution of cells and bottles are loaded in. It can process 120 samples per hour.

severe liver disease PT and APTT will both be prolonged; it is unusual for the TT to be affected.

You will come across a lot of patients taking anti-coagulants, most frequently warfarin, which has a long half-life and is taken orally. This is used to prevent clots in patients who have had a deep vein thrombosis and pulmonary embolus and as primary prevention for patients at risk for several reasons, most commonly atrial fibrillation. Heparin is used in hospital for rapid anticoagulation of patients who have thrombosis. It has to be given subcutaneously or intra venously; it has a very short half-life and is therefore easily controlled. Warfarin therapy is monitored using the PT, Heparin with the APTT. The PT is expressed as the international normalized ratio (INR) which is the ratio of the patient's PT over the mean of the PT reference range using an international sensitivity index. This makes the result more standardized for comparison purposes.

Warfarin is the most commonly used anti-coagulant. An INR result of 2 means that the patient's blood will take twice as long to clot than the control.

Causes of Anaemia

1. Iron deficiency

2. Chronic inflammation or infection (anaemia of chronic disease)

3. Blood loss

4. Deficiency of B_{12} or folate

5. Deficiency of erythropoietin (most chronic renal failure)

6. Increased RBC destruction (haemolytic anaemias)

7. Marrow failure (aplastic, usually toxic drugs or radio therapy)

8. Malignant disease in marrow (leukaemia, myeloma)

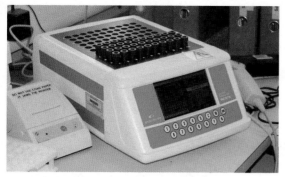

Machine for measuring ESR in the tubes

Patients who need anticoagulation have differing target values depending on their condition. Those who are taking it because they have atrial fibrillation or have had a recent deep vein thrombosis will have a target value of between 2 and 3 whereas those who have a mechanical heart valve replacement are at higher risk and will have a higher therapeutic range of between 3 and 4. We receive a large number of referrals for dental extractions for patients on warfarin but it has been shown repeatedly that if the INR is below 4 then if they are managed correctly with the sockets sutured and packed with oxidised cellulose gauze, then post extraction bleeding is no more of a problem than patients not on warfarin. If the INR is above 4 then this is outside the therapeutic range and the patients should see their GP to have their dose adjusted before the extractions.

Erythrocyte Sedimentation Rate and C Reactive Protein

Erythrocyte sedimentation rate (ESR) is a simple test in which anti-coagulated blood is left for the red cells to sediment to the bottom of a tube. The result is expressed in the number of millimetres the red cells fall in an hour. The ESR will be increased in disease processes that increase certain plasma proteins, which cause aggregation of the red cells and in certain anaemias where the number of red cells is decreased. ESR is normally 1 – 10 mms/hour in males and 5-10 mms/hour in females. This increases with age by about 0.8 mms per 5 years. ESR is a very unspecific test; it is raised in pregnancy, where there is significant tissue damage, infection, malignancy and in certain individuals with no disease. A decrease in ESR is uncommon and usually of little clinical significance; it occurs in polycythaemia.

C reactive protein (CRP) is present normally in low concentration in the plasma and is a more modern non-specific test as an alternative to ESR. It is increased in inflammation, infection and malignancy, but is not affected by red cell numbers.

ESR and CRP are used to monitor treatment responses to patients with complicated and extensive disease processes e.g. inflammatory or infective.

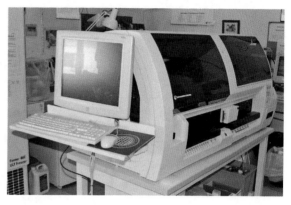

Coagulation analyser

38. <u>Blood Tests - Biochemistry</u>

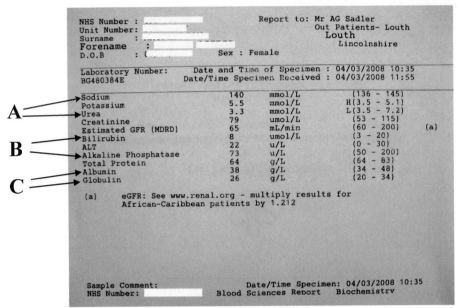

Standard Biochemistry results form

A. Urea and electrolytes (Us & Es) Sodium (Na$^+$), and Potassium (K$^+$) have been traditionally requested and analysed together. Nowadays, however, the analysing equipment will process multiple biochemical and immunological assays simultaneously on one sample.

Na$^+$ is the primary electrolyte in the blood; hypernatraemia may be due to a very high salt intake or dehydration from inadequate fluid intake or excessive fluid loss from sweating or diarrhoea. Na$^+$ concentration may be low in excessive fluid retention. Neither of these situations are of much relevance to us in everyday OMFS where, should we encounter patients with severe electrolyte or fluid balance abnormality, we would request the assistance of a physician.

Hyperkalaemia may be due to renal disease or diabetes. Hypokalaemia may be due to excessive K$^+$ loss in diarrhoea or from excessive loss due to diuretic medication. As surgeons our main concern with abnormal K$^+$ concentration will be the potential effect on cardiac muscle. Severe hyperkalaemia can result in instability of the cardiac muscle leading to cardiac arrest and in hypokalaemia cardiac arrhythmias may occur. We would therefore wish to test for K$^+$ concentration for any patient receiving a general

anaesthetic if they have renal disease, poorly controlled diabetes or are taking diuretics. In general a narrow reference range for a blood test indicates potentially serious consequences when it is either too high or low and this is the case with potassium.

Urea is a waste product of normal metabolism. There is a gradual increase in the blood concentration with age due to gradual decline of renal function. Urea may be increased in more advanced renal disease but not early on. It may also be increased in starvation and dehydration.

Creatinine is a waste product more specifically of muscle metabolism. Raised creatinine will be a more sensitive marker for early renal disease.

Estimated Glomerular Filtration Rate (eGFR) is calculated from the MDRD (Modification of Diet in Renal Disease study) formula; this includes creatinine level, age, sex and ethnicity. If the estimated glomerular filtration rate (eGFR) is decreased further investigation may be needed for chronic kidney disease. If a low eGFR is found on routine testing we should alert the patient's GP to deal with this later.

B. Bilirubin, alanine transferase (ALT) and alkaline phosphatase are together known as the liver

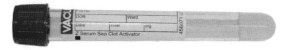

Combined clinical chemistry and immunology is tested on serum. Blood is taken into a tube which contains a gel, with silica in it; this activates coagulation. The tube is centrifuged to separate the serum; the gel moves up forming a barrier between serum and fibrin

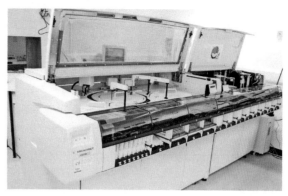

The Abbott Architest integrated general chemistry & immunoassay analyser will process 1200 clinical chemistry and 200 immunoassays per hour. Only one serum specimen is needed for both.

function tests (LFTs). Bilirubin is derived from haemoglobin breakdown and is increased in liver disease, where there is obstruction to bile flow and in haemolytic anaemias where there is increased breakdown of red cells. If it is very high the patient may be clinically jaundiced. Alanine transferase and alkaline phosphatase are metabolic catalysts in liver cells. They are released into the blood stream, where they have no function, when liver cells are damaged and hence their presence usually indicates liver disease. However they are present in other tissues, notably the pancreas, kidney, heart and muscle. Alkaline phosphatase is present in osteoclasts and will be released into the plasma in any condition where there is high osteoclastic activity. This will include childhood growth spurts, Paget's disease of bone, healing fractures and bone cancer including metastatic disease. We may therefore wish to order these tests when a patient has a history of liver disease and is to receive an anaesthetic or if they have cancer and we want to know if metastatic disease has affected liver function or we wish to know if there might be bone involvement.

C. Albumin and globulin together make up the plasma proteins. Albumin is the more abundant, being about 60%; it is synthesised in the liver from amino acids. It acts as a transport medium for water insoluble substances in the blood and is important in maintaining blood plasma volume. Albumin may be low in chronic liver disease (cirrhosis) but not in acute; this will lead to increased fluid in the interstitial spaces and possibly oedema. It may be reduced in malnutrition due to inadequate amino acid intake or in severe burns. It will be raised in patients who are dehydrated. We will want to know the albumin level for new patients who present with advanced mouth cancer as they may have a low albumin from inadequate nutrition. Globulins make up the rest of the plasma proteins; they include the gamma globulins which are antibodies and they act as enzymes and carriers. They may be elevated in chronic infections and renal disease and may be decreased in renal disease which leads to protein loss, haemolytic anaemia, liver disease and hypogammaglobulinaemia

127

39. <u>Blood Tests - Immunology</u>

These are used infrequently in OMFS. However, we may occasionally test for antinuclear antibodies (ANA) in a patient with a dry mouth who we suspect may have Sjögren's syndrome (SS). ANA are raised in a variety of conditions such as systemic lupus, rheumatoid arthritis and chronic active hepatitis. About 70% of patients with SS will have raised titres of ANA. These are expressed as the dilution at which they may be detected; normal is 1:40. In addition 70% of SS patients will have a raised titre of the ANA sub types Anti SS-A (also known as anti-Ro) and 40% will have a raised titre of Anti SS-B (known as anti-La). Rheumatoid factor is also likely to be raised in 60% of these patients. The significance of SS (apart from the dry mouth) is that there is an increased incidence of low grade lymphoma and this may be associated with a low level of complement C4.

Immunoglobulins may be tested in patients who have repeated infections. IgM will be raised in patients who have significant acute inflammation. IgE may be of help in supporting a diagnosis of an allergy. However, the normal range is very wide and it is possible to have a raised specific IgE against a single allergen when total IgE is normal; thus it is of limited use. Occasionally we see a patient with recurrent oedematous swelling around the face. A rare cause of this is hereditary angio-oedema due to complement C1 inhibitor deficiency. Patients with these clinical symptoms should have their complement C4 tested as a screening test. If this is normal then they will not have heredity angio-oedema and there is no need to test for complement C1 inhibitor levels.

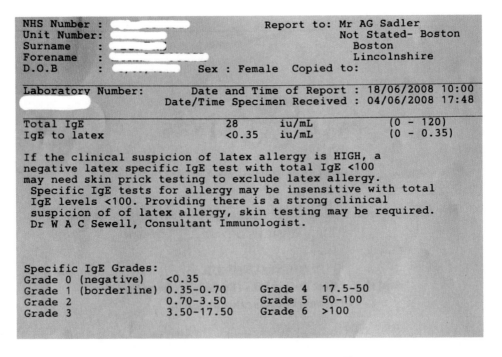

Immunology report for suspected latex allergy

40. <u>Understanding Fluid and Blood Replacement</u>

Humans can last only a few days without adequate water intake. The consequence of dehydration may include headache, hypotension, dizziness, fainting, delirium, loss of consciousness and ultimately death. Signs of dehydration will include dryness of the mouth, loss of skin elasticity, decreased or no urine output (should be 60 mls. per hour), hypotension on standing and increased cardiac and respiratory rate.

In OMFS we frequently need to give fluid intravenously for patients unable to take it by mouth. Usually this is because they are having surgery for which they need to be starved. Sometimes we see patients who are dehydrated; most commonly this is because they have been drinking alcohol (which is a diuretic) and have sustained a broken jaw.

The other fluid which our patients may need replacing is blood. This may be due to heavy blood loss in trauma but more usually is likely to be as a result of loss during surgery. Inadequate blood volume is called hypovolaemia, the symptoms may be nausea, thirst and dizziness. Signs may be increased pulse, decreased blood pressure and decreased peripheral perfusion which is seen as delayed capillary refill on pressing the skin. Eventually there may be confusion, loss of consciousness, heart failure and death. It is unusual for OMF surgeons to have to administer blood

Compartment	Vol. in 70 kg. man	Na$^+$	K$^+$	
Intracellular	30 L	low	high	Insulin drives K into cells
Interstitial	9 L	high	low	
Intravascular	3 L	high	low	Higher protein than interstitial + blood cells

Fluid compartment properties

themselves as the acutely injured patient will already have been dealt with by the Accident and Emergency doctors, and during surgery it will be given by the anaesthetist. However it will do no harm to know the principles.

There are basically three types of fluids which can be transfused intravenously; these are crystalloids, colloids and blood products, usually packed red cells. Crystalloids are of low molecular weight; they pass freely across cell membranes and, when given intravenously, will pass from the intravascular to

Input	Amount (mls)	Loss	Amount (mls)
Oral fluid	1300	Urine	1500
		Stools	200
In food	900	Lungs	300
Oxidation	300	Skin	500
Total	2500	Total	2500

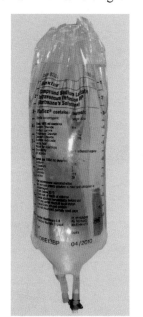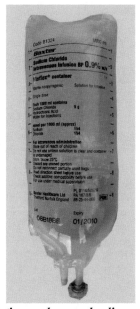

Crystalloids Hartman's solution and normal saline

Daily fluid input and loss average 70kg. male

Fluid	Property	Distributes	Use
5% Glucose	Isotonic with plasma. Glucose is metabolised so is effectively just water	Distributed throughout whole body-water	Crystalloid. Provides fluid & nothing else
Hartman's solution (compound sodium lactate)	Isotonic, is water with Na^+ K^+ Ca^{++} Cl^- & Lactic acid	As above	Crystalloid. Provides fluid & electrolytes, more physiological
0.9% NaCl (normal saline)	Contains 150 mmols/L Na^+	Throughout extracellular fluid only as Na^+ is excluded from intracellular fluid	Crystalloid. Provides fluid and Na^+
Hydrolysed gelatin solutions _(e.g. Gelofusine®, Haemaccel®)_	High molecular weight gelatin which is metabolised & excreted over a few hours. Contains Na^+ Cl^- OH^- Anaphylaxis can occur	Initially stays in vascular compartment but is distributed into extracellular fluid as gelatin is metabolised	Colloid, expands plasma volume after blood loss
Hydroxyethyl starch (_Voluven®_)	High molecular weight starch, is metabolised but less quickly than gelatin. Contains Na^+ Cl^- OH^-	Stays in vascular compartment but longer than gelatin.	Colloid, expands plasma volume after blood loss. Less allergenic than gelatin
Blood	Packed cells collected from donated blood. Only fluid which carries 0_2	Only in vascular compartment	Loss of blood where Hb is dropping significantly

**Commonly used IV fluids (there are many others especially those used in special situations)**

interstitial fluid and then into cells. Crystalloids are cheap and without side effects; examples include dextrose solution, normal saline and Hartman's solution (which is preferred by physicians because it is more physiological). The dextrose in the solutions is of no nutritional value; it is there to make the water isotonic. Crystalloids are what we give our patients who cannot take fluid by mouth for whatever reason. It will also be the first fluid given to patients who have lost blood before colloid is given. A special note about normal (isotonic) saline: it will pass from the blood into the interstitial space but will largely be kept out of the intracellular space because Na^+ is actively pumped out in exchange for K^+.

Colloids are of high molecular weight; they do not dissolve or pass easily through cell membranes. They can be used when the intravascular fluid needs replacement consequent upon blood loss. They can increase osmotic pressure and may leak across membranes causing oedema, and occasionally they cause anaphylactic reactions. They include gelatin and starch. Gelatins are the most frequently used colloids (_Haemaccel®_ & _Gelofusine®_). The colloids, due to their higher molecular weight, will stay in the intravascular compartment until the gelatin or starch is metabolised. When gelatin is metabolised, within a few hours, the fluid will then move from the intravascular compartment into the interstitial and eventually intracellular space. However, starches (_Voluven®_) take about 17 days to be metabolised rather than the few hours taken by gelatin, so the fluid stays in the vessels longer. Starch is therefore becoming more popular and it is thought to provoke fewer anaphylactic reactions.

Blood (packed cells) will remain in the vessels. The reason for giving it rather than colloid is to maintain the oxygen carrying capacity of the blood. Blood transfusion has many potential complications

United Lincolnshire Hospitals **NHS** NHS Trust

Chart No. (1) 2 3 4 5   **No. charts in use** 1 2 3 4 5

Notes:
1. Bolus intravenous injections should be prescribed on the main drug chart
2. If an additive is to be used are you sure that: it needs to be given intravenously it is compatible with the fluid
3. If no additive is required strike through, or write 'NIL'

DRUG SENSITIVITIES

No	
Source	
Height	182 cm Weight 81 kg
BSA	m² BMI

...AILS

Na: U (57
M   i
Da 14 (ROAD
NEWARK
Ho: NOTTINGHAMSHIRE
NG DOB Ot .87
NH NHS 60

Ward CLAYTON   Consultant SAYLER.

PRESCRIPTION							ADMINISTRATION					
Date	Start time	Intravenous fluid	Volume	Additive & dose	Duration infusion	Rate	Signature V Number & bleep / ext.	Date started	Time started	Started by	Checked by	Time finished	Volume given
6/9/08	22.00	5% dextrose	1 l		8 hrs		Hade.	6/9	22.05	Je	Sw	06.00	1 l
7/9/0	6.00	5% dextrose	1 l		8 hrs		Hade.	7/9	100	Je			
7/9/0	16.00	Normal saline	1 l		8		A Sodley						

__Fluid Prescription Chart.__ Each bag of fluid is prescribed sequentially. The boxes on the right are for the nurse to record that it has been given. This is a suitable regime for a 24 hour period for a fit adult who is taking no fluid by mouth. Increase the amount to a litre every 6 hours if they are dehydrated (as from drinking alcohol) or pyrexial. If too much fluid is given it will be passed harmlessly as urine. Do not give fluid fast to an elderly patient or someone with heart disease as it could tip them into cardiac failure. If after two days the patient is still taking fluids IV then add 40 mols. of K^+ to each bag in the additive column.

and side effects, which include mild transfusion reactions (common), severe haemolytic reactions, sepsis, HIV or hepatitis transmission and lung injury. We therefore keep transfusion to a minimum. During surgery, depending upon the fitness of the patient, generally half of the blood volume can be lost before it is necessary to transfuse with blood.

Blood loss is initially replaced with crystalloid (usually Hartman's solution) and then colloid; we use starch (*Voluven*®). The haemoglobin level is then monitored during surgery using a haemoglobin analyser (*HemoCue*®) and transfusion started when the level drops significantly. The haemoglobin level at which transfusion is started will depend upon a number of factors, which include the patient's pre-operative level, their age and cardiovascular fitness. For a fit person with a normal pre-operative level it can drop to 8 or even lower but in an elderly person with ischaemic heart disease a safer level will be about 10.

So, having discussed the theory, what of prescribing fluids for patients on the ward? If you read

a textbook of medicine or surgery you will find that it can be very complicated. Fluid replacement will depend upon what fluid may have been lost and how. It may be lost as a result of vomiting, diarrhoea, blood loss, renal disease, exudates from burns, etc. It will also depend upon the amount lost, as recorded on a fluid balance chart, and the patient's renal function. However in OMFS we are usually dealing with patients who are generally fit and have normal kidneys; this makes it very simple.

The most likely, if not the only, circumstance in which you will be asked to prescribe fluid will be for a patient who cannot take fluid by mouth. They will need only water so you will need to write up only a crystalloid. Thus you can prescribe a dextrose solution

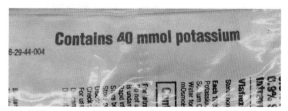

__Fluid bags are available with potassium added__

and add some saline for their daily Na$^+$ needs (approx. 120 to 140 mmols. per day). In the unlikely event that the patient needs fluids for more than two days you should add some K$^+$ (approx. 60 mmols. per day). Prescribe as on the fluid chart illustrated. If the patient is dehydrated from drinking alcohol or is pyrexial (which leads to a greater insensible fluid loss), increase the amount; they will come to no harm if you give a little too much as they will pass it off as urine. However if you have an elderly patient with a compromised heart you could put them into heart failure if too much fluid is given too rapidly. If prescribing fluid in the emergency situation you should start with Hartman's solution or saline, as rehydrating a patient with dextrose or dextrose saline carries a risk of producing hyponatraemia which can be dangerous. The electrolytes should normally be checked daily for a patient on IV fluids.

The most commonly used blood products are packed red cells, platelets, fresh frozen plasma and cryoprecipitate (which contains fibrinogen, factor 8, Von Willibrand factor and factor).

When we say we are transfusing blood we mean we are using packed red cells with no plasma, clotting factors or other cells. The purpose is to increase oxygen carriage; there is no artificial substitute which will do this. We can use colloids to expand blood volume. In OMFS we are likely to transfuse only if there has been significant blood loss, either as a result of major trauma or major surgery, usually a cancer resection.

Donated blood is processed into its constituents to use separately, so should a patient undergoing surgery be thrombocytopenic we would request platelets. We would ask for fresh frozen plasma if the patient is bleeding and is short of clotting factors; most usually this would be if they have had massive bleeding and have been transfused a lot of red cells. There are boxes on the request form (or on screen) to ask for platelets or fresh frozen plasma. Always request a full blood count at the same time as you will need a base line measurement of the haemoglobin.

The laboratory will test the sample for blood grouping using the ABO and Rhesus systems and then take donated red cells of the same compatible group and test them against serum from the patient's sample (cross match). In order to facilitate this they will want to know if the blood group is already known and if the patient has had any previous transfusions or has been

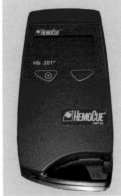

The HemoCue® haemoglobin analyser is kept in the operating theatre. It can produce a result within a few minutes on a blood sample taken from a thumb prick. The result is claimed to be as accurate as that from a venous sample assayed in the laboratory.

pregnant as either of these may predispose to antibody formation.

If we know we will need blood in advance, for example for planned major cancer surgery, we will tick the box on the request form for blood to be cross matched: we will say how many units we anticipate we will need and when we need it. Blood will then be cross matched and kept in the refrigerator to be collected. If we think we might need blood but are not definitely sure then the lab will not want to cross match. In this case you will tick the box to 'group and save'. This means the blood is tested for the group using ABO and Rhesus systems and the patient's serum is saved in the fridge to be used to cross match should they get a phone call from the operating theatre to say blood is needed.

You may find that the laboratory will prefer to receive a sample a week or so before to test for ABO and Rhesus grouping and to test for atypical antibodies, so that they are forewarned, and then another sample on the day of operation for cross matching.

You should be aware that when a patient receives blood it invariably leads to some pyrexia. Although the donated blood had been found to be compatible using the ABO and Rhesus systems and cross matched there is always some degree of immunological reaction to it.

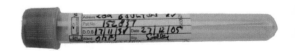

An EDTA containing tube is used for transfusion testing. Always hand write the details on the tube.

41. Prescribing Medication in the Hospital

When you start to work in the hospital you will have to prescribe a few medications which will be unfamiliar to you and use prescription forms that you will not be used to. However the number of drugs that we use in OMFS is small. This is, of course, apart from drugs for inpatients that they have been taking prior to their hospital admission.

You will almost certainly find that the team you work for has a policy concerning which drugs to use and if not there will be a normal accepted practice that you will soon get used to. You should prescribe only a few drugs that you will become familiar with. Always check in the British National Formulary (BNF) when you first use a medication and subsequently if you are uncertain about interactions with medication the patient may already be taking.

You will not be able to prescribe any drug you like. There will be a hospital formulary of drugs that have been approved for use in the hospital. In most hospitals this can be accessed, like all hospital policies and procedures, on the intranet. Every hospital trust will have a drug and therapeutics committee which manages the introduction of new drugs. Their approvals come from recommendations from Consultants after consideration of evidence of efficacy from the literature, cost and availability of other medication with the same purpose. The committee will tend to follow the recommendations of the National Institute for Heath & Care Excellence (NICE).

Outpatient scripts should be on a standard hospital outpatient prescription form which must be taken to the hospital pharmacy to be dispensed. Some clinics will prescribe on peach coloured FP10HP forms which can be taken to an outside chemist. The cost of drugs is then recharged to the hospital so these forms are discouraged by not having them freely available in most hospital areas.

You should only issue a script for the minimal medication needed before the patient can get to their GP for a repeat prescription and in any case no longer than 28 days. This is because the GPs hold the funding for outpatient medication.

In the unlikely event that you need to prescribe a controlled drug you should specify the generic name of the drug, the dose, total quantity in words and

262504

THIS PRESCRIPTION CAN ONLY BE DISPENSED IN THE HOSPITAL

Outpatient Prescription Sheet | AFFIX ADDRESSOGRAPH

United Lincolnshire Hospitals NHS
Headquarters Address:
County Hospital
Greetwell Road
Lincoln
Lincs. LN2 4AX

U 02
M   1
2. ____ ROAD
SKEGNESS
LINCOLNSHIRE
P   DOB .   53
NHS 4   67
(1st Unit no U   69)

Drug Sensitivities		NHS Number	
Age if under 12	Weight	Date of Birth	
		Consultant	SADLER

Medicine (Approved Name), Dose and Directions | Dispensing details

℞ IBUPROFEN   400mgm
×3 daily   3 day   (9)
please

30 days or the nearest original pack, will be provided unless a shorter course is requested.

| Signature of Prescriber A Sadler | Date 20/2/09. | Payment details |
| Prescriber's Name and Initials in BLOCK Capitals SADLER | Contact Ext: | Bleep: |

Outpatient prescribing will be very similar to what you are already used to. You should clearly indicate the identity of the drug using the generic name, the dose, route of administration, frequency and duration.

figures written in ink. If using an addressograph label sign it to prevent a new one being put on top of it. Add your signature and print your name.

Prescribing for inpatients should be on the standard inpatient prescription charts which consist of a folder with four pages. There is a different page for drugs given once only, regular medication and drugs to be given only when needed. There will be additional charts for prescribing intravenous fluids, insulin, anticoagulants as well as charts for drugs administered by a syringe driver and total parenteral nutrition which you will not be involved with.

Many patients coming into hospital will already be on some medication; this needs to be prescribed on the chart. The patient and medication will be assessed by the nurse and most will be able to take their own drugs themselves without having to have them dispensed by the nurse. This is called Self-Administered Medication.

Other medication will be dispensed by the patient's nurse at standard times and she will sign on the patient's chart to show that it has been given. Note that the times on the charts do not exactly fit into a convenient division of the day into 6 or 8 hours for drugs given x4 or x3 per day but represent a working compromise.

Each day a pharmacist will visit the ward and check each patient's drug chart. They will ensure that the medication is in stock in the ward drug cabinet and in sufficient quantity. They will also check the dose, frequency of administration and any interactions with other medication. This is a very valuable service as it provides a safeguard in the prevention of errors. You should put your bleep or extension number next to the prescription so that you can be easily contacted if there is a problem.

Antibiotic prescribing should be kept to the absolute minimum in order to reduce antimicrobial resistance, particularly MRSA and Clostridium Difficile. Every hospital will have an antibiotic policy which should be followed. For example you may have to get the permission of a Consultant microbiologist before you can prescribe a cephalosporin, which you may want to do if a patient is allergic to penicillin.

Antibiotics should only be prescribed for a maximum

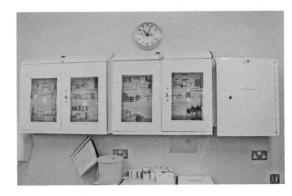

Stock drug cabinets in the treatment room on the ward. The contents are displayed by a photograph on the door. There is a separate cabinet for controlled drugs and a paper copy of the hospital formulary to refer to.

of five days, except for certain specific infections. Strictly speaking they should be prescribed after the infecting organism has been identified by sampling and culturing and the antibiotic sensitivity defined in the laboratory. However, in practice it may often be the case that we need to prescribe before this is known and by the time the result is expected the need has passed as the antibiotic should be stopped as soon as possible. The mere presence of an infection is not necessarily an indication for antibiotics. Most oral infection, particularly of dental origin, will be adequately managed by removing the cause, draining pus and allowing the patient's immune system to deal with the rest.

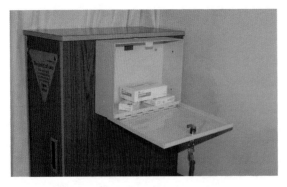

The patient's medication will be kept in a locked cabinet adjacent to the patient's bed. The patient will have the key for it and a nurse will hold a master key for all the cabinets on the ward.

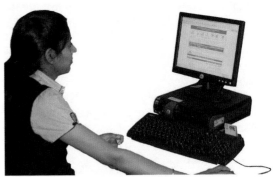

Medication to take home is likely to be prescribed on the computer with a digital signature, note the personal identity card slotted into the top right of the keyboard necessary to identify the prescriber. Increasingly hospitals are developing paperless clinical records for all inpatients drug prescriptions which are made on-line on the clinical records system

Ward drug chart Page 1 of 4

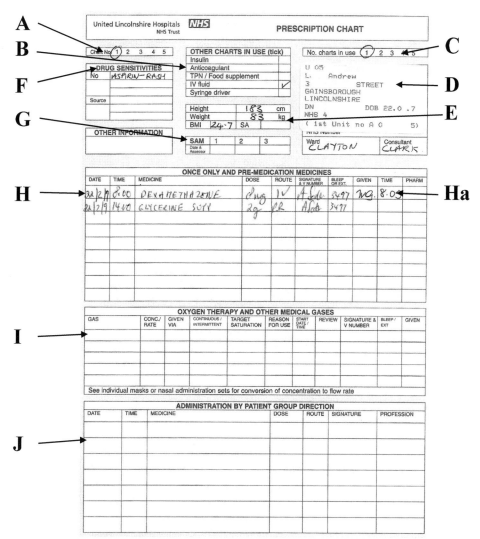

A: The number of this particular chart (Patients in hospital for a while may have accumulated several consecutive charts.) B: Special charts that may be in use C: Total number of charts in use for this patient (Usually there is only one.) D: Demographic details of the patient, addressograph label, ward and Consultant details

E: Height, weight, body mass index and surface area. This may have a bearing on drug dosage.

F: Known drug allergies and sensitivities G: Self administered medication, number of medications the patient takes themselves and who has assessed their capability to do this and the date H: Prescription for drugs given once only rather than those taken on a recurring basis Ha: Signed and timed by nurse when drug is given

I: Oxygen and gases. We are very unlikely to use this unless we have a patient with severe chronic obstructive pulmonary disease (COPD) or a bad post-operative chest infection. J: Drugs prescribed by nurses under a 'group direction' where they are permitted to prescribe certain drugs in certain circumstances according to a protocol.

Ward drug chart Page 2 & 3 of 4 (part). Regular prescriptions

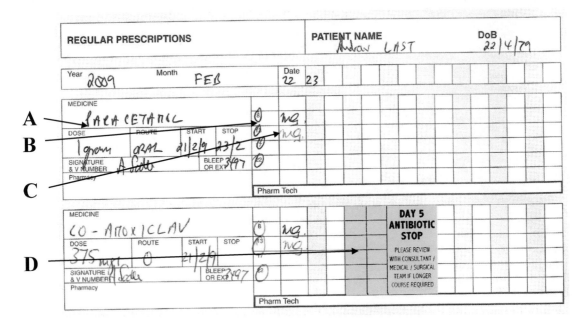

A: *The prescribed drug, route of administration, start & stop date, the signature of the prescriber & contact bleep or extension number for the pharmacist to contact them if there is any problem* **B:** *Standard times of drug rounds for the medication to be given* **C:** *Signature of nurse when dose given* **D:** *5 day stop sticker placed by the pharmacist. This is placed automatically so that antibiotics are not continued beyond the minimum time needed.*

Ward drug chart . As Required prescriptions

A: *The prescribed drug, its reason for use, signature of the prescriber & contact bleep or extension number* **B:** *Dose, route, frequency it can be administered and maximum dose in 24 hours* **C:** *Signature of nurse when dose given, dose and time*

42. <u>Understanding the Anaesthetist</u>

The first thing to be said about anaesthetics is that they should be avoided if possible. Modern anaesthetics have never been safer but they are not as safe as no anaesthetic. Using general anaesthesia has never been more expensive. Anaesthetists only wish to give general anaesthetic in the operating theatre, which is the most costly facility in the hospital, another reason to carry out as much surgery as possible using local anaesthetic outside the operating theatre. In our hospital it is now quite rare for a patient to be anaesthetised for a dento-alveolar procedure; we simply do not offer it. Nearly all cases can be done with local, or local and sedation. There are a few exceptions, such as the IV drug abuser who may be difficult to sedate.

Anaesthetists provide a number of different services apart from giving general anaesthetics. They provide a pain relief service for obstetrics, run a chronic pain service for outpatients, supervise the nurse-provided acute pain service for inpatients, and they also run the Intensive Care Unit and provide a sedation service.

Anaesthetists carry out some sedation for us for patients who have severely compromised general health, such as ischaemic heart disease or chronic obstructive pulmonary disease. In this circumstance the safest way to deal with them is to use local anaesthetic in the operating theatre with an anaesthetist monitoring them with an ECG, administering a small amount of sedation intravenously and oxygen via a small nasal cannula. Fit patients who are having minor surgery and are ASA grade 1 or 2, we may sedate ourselves with midazolam in the outpatient clinic.

The anaesthetist will be responsible for the patient's systemic well being whilst in the operating theatre. He will normally visit the patient pre-operatively to ensure they are to fit for anaesthetic, to discuss the anaesthetic with the patient and to make themselves cognizant of any special problems the patient may have. They will administer the anaesthetic in the anaesthetic room, then transfer the patient to the theatre where they will monitor the anaesthetic and the patient's general condition.

During surgery the anaesthetist will administer any intravenous medication that may be requested, for example antibiotics or steroids to prevent swelling (usually dexamethasone 8mgs), and will be in charge of the same. You must ask the anaesthetist's

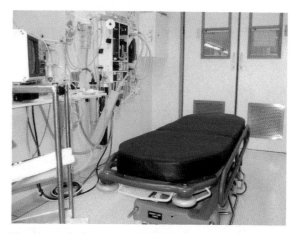

The anaesthetic room will have all the anaesthetic equipment of the theatre itself

permission if you wish to give any medication at the operation site, for example local anaesthetic and vasoconstrictor to increase pain control or decrease bleeding. At the end of the operation the patient will be woken up by the anaesthetist and accompanied to the recovery room where they will be looked after by a recovery nurse. Throughout, the anaesthetist will still be in charge of the patient's general condition, and will give permission when the patient has recovered sufficiently for them to be transferred back to the ward with their named nurse.

A trained anaesthetic nurse or an operating department practitioner (ODP) will assist by fetching and carrying, drawing up drugs with the surgeon, and occasionally monitoring the patient, particularly during a long case. In some hospitals, there are 'physician's assistants' who can give the whole anaesthetic supervised by an anaesthetist who might be elsewhere in the theatre suite.

You will find that some specialize in one area of practice, particularly chronic pain or intensive care. More frequently they will have a special interest and skill in some particular practice, such as children or OMFS. In our speciality we are always operating in the area where the anaesthetist wants to be in control of the patient's airway, which has its own special problems, and small children should be anaesthetised by someone who has had special training and a continued special interest in dealing with children. We frequently operate on children under two years for dog bites and other lacerations to the face.

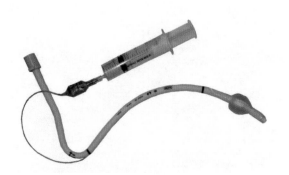

The endotrachael tube prepared for the anaesthetist by the ODP. It has a cuff which is inflated with air from a syringe to make a seal within the trachea.

When the anaesthetist visits the patient before the beginning of the operating list he will expect to know exactly what the surgeon intends to do. Usually this will be obvious from the operating list, particularly if the surgeon and anaesthetist usually work together on similar cases. However they should be informed if anything out of the ordinary is contemplated, such as length of the surgery or special airway requirements. Any pre-operative investigations needed should have been organised at a pre-booking or pre-admission clinic by nurses according to agreed protocols, and all patients receiving a general anaesthetic for all but in 'emergency' operations should have no solid food for six hours pre-operatively and no fluids for four hours to ensure their stomachs are empty, in order to minimise the risk of aspiration of stomach contents into the airway. In some hospitals patients having major or complicated surgery and those with complex medical problems who might be high risk may be required to see the anaesthetist in addition to the nurse led clinic.

One of the anaesthetist's responsibilities is the patient's airway and he will usually place a pack in the pharynx at the beginning of the surgery to catch blood or other debris. The pack remains the responsibility of the anaesthetist and at the end of the operation the surgeon should ask the anaesthetist if he wants his pack removed. When the reply is a certainty it should be removed and the pharynx sucked out. This should include careful suction of the post nasal space under direct vision or blood clots caused by bleeding during nasal intubation. The anaesthetist will normally check the pharynx themselves using a laryngoscope before they wake the patient up. One of the questions that the anaesthetist is likely to ask before the surgery is what sort of tube you want. He

is referring to the tube in which he delivers the anaesthetic gases to the lungs and, as you will almost certainly be operating around the mouth and face, a mask over the nose and mouth will be contra-indicated as it will obstruct your access. There are four possibilities – the first is an endotracheal tube passed through the nose and known as a 'nasal tube'. This will be the most convenient for operating in the mouth as it will obviously not interfere with your access to the operative site.

From the anaesthetic point of view it does have the disadvantage in that it is not so easily passed and this may become a problem if you are operating on a child or somebody with a narrow nasal airway, particularly somebody who has a deviated septum, allergic rhinitis or a history of trauma to the nose. In these circumstances it may be easier to compromise and work with the second option - an endotracheal tube passed through the mouth known as an 'oral tube'. It is quite usual to carry out many procedures in the mouth around an oral tube, particularly unilateral ones, although it does require some adaption for the surgeon. Some procedures are not possible with an oral tube, such as reduction and fixation of fractures where you will need to occlude the teeth together during the operation. The third possibility is a laryngeal mask. Here the anaesthetic gas is passed through a rather thicker tube and the seal with the airway is made at the larynx by contact with a fairly bulky mask apparatus. From the anaesthetic point of view it does away with the need to pass a tube through the larynx into the trachea so the patient does not require paralysing and the anaesthetic process is much quicker. From the operative point of view the tube is quite bulky and difficult to work round and if you are not used to working with a laryngeal mask it is quite possible that you may dislodge it during the procedure. However, an experienced surgeon can frequently work adequately around a laryngeal mask which has been expertly placed.

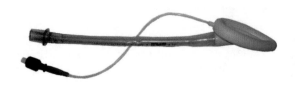

Laryngeal mask airway (LMA)

Lastly the anaesthetic can be delivered through a tracheostomy. This is reserved for our major head and neck cancer patients and those with severe facial trauma. The patient is anaesthetised in the conventional manner and an oral tube placed, then a tracheostomy is made and a tube passed into the trachea as the anaesthetist withdraws the oral tube. Now the surgeon can operate anywhere in the head and neck without compromising the airway and is secure in the knowledge that the airway will not be affected by post-operative swelling or bleeding.

Once in the anaesthetic room the anaesthetist will again check the patient's wrist band and ask the patient to confirm their identity. The anaesthetic can then commence. The first task is to place an IV cannula; the ODP will have drawn up all the drugs needed into syringes and labelled them. The anaesthetic is usually induced with an intravenous infusion of an anaesthetic drug such as Propofol. Sometimes the patient may be induced by breathing an inhalation anaesthetic through a mask. Once consciousness is lost the patient will be ventilated with a face mask using an inhalation anaesthetic carried in a mixture of nitrous oxide and oxygen. Once they are deep enough a muscle relaxant is given and a tube passed. The tube is then connected to the anaesthetic machine and secured. The patient's eyes are covered to prevent accidental injury.

Once the patient is anaesthetised there are other preparations to make before they are ready for surgery. For major cases this may include an arterial line to directly measure blood pressure and to sample for blood gases and pH levels, a central venous pressure line to help gauge fluid status and a cerebral function monitor to measure the depth of the anaesthetic. Once the anaesthetic has been administered the patient will be transferred to the operating theatre where they will be connected to a blood pressure cuff and a pulse oximeter. There may be a urinary catheter to monitor urine output and a temperature probe (often in the urinary catheter) to measure core body temperature. A naso-gastric tube may be passed to aspirate stomach secretions and prevent regurgitation. The patient may be covered in an inflatable blanket to maintain their temperature and have pneumatic compression stockings to gently squeeze their calves to prevent thrombosis in the large veins in the legs. This can be fatal if a clot should embolise and pass into the lungs.

A more recent development is the Total Intravenous Anaesthetic (TIVA). Here the propofol used for induction is continued, using a syringe driver

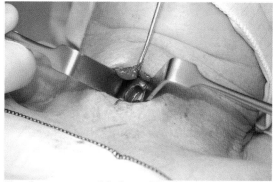

Tracheostomy and below with Portex tube in position

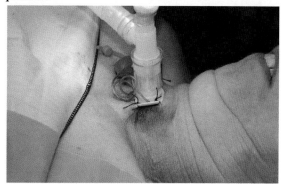

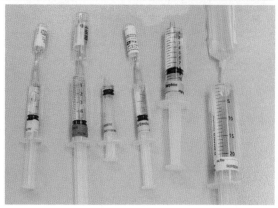

Drugs drawn up and labelled by the ODP. From left: Dexamethasone (steroid to reduce swelling & anti emetic), Mivacurium (short acting non depolarising muscle relaxant), Atropine (antimuscarinic), Ondansetron (anti-emetic), Morphine (opiate analgesic), Co-amoxiclav (antibiotic)

throughout the operation. This may be accompanied by a continuous infusion of a short acting opiate such as remifentanil. In this technique the only gas delivered to the patient's lungs is a mixture of oxygen and air.

During surgery the anaesthetist and ODP will monitor the patient and record the progress on the anaesthetic chart. They will administer any drugs and at the end will wake the patient up and accompany them to the recovery room, handing their care over to the recovery nurse. The patient remains the anaesthetist's responsibility while they are still in the theatre suite. The recovery nurse will ask the anaesthetist's permission to send the patient back to the ward when they have recovered sufficiently. The anaesthetist will ensure that the patient has post-operative analgesia prescribed for the post-operative period; they regard this as one of their responsibilities and are normally very keen that we inject a long acting local anaesthetic with a vasoconstrictor around the operation site as it contributes to a more comfortable recovery.

We have already mentioned that in much OMFS we are attempting to share the upper airway with the anaesthetist. This can cause potential difficulties. In addition there will be a number of specific problems related to our patients which might cause difficulty with conventional intubation. The anaesthetist will want to be forewarned of these so that he can modify his technique. These include patients with obstruction to the airway as a result of cancer or trauma, abnormality of anatomy such as severe retrognathia, limitation of jaw opening consequent upon jaw ankylosis, and fractures of the mandible, maxilla or malar. A common problem is limited mouth opening caused by an acute dental abscess which has been allowed to prosper by negligent management with antibiotics rather than by early drainage by pulp extirpation or extraction.

The anaesthetist will always assess the difficulty or ease of intubation before starting. This assessment will involve an examination of the patient's neck. Difficulty can be anticipated in patients with short, fat necks and those with reduced neck flexion as might be caused by arthritis. They will assess jaw movement in an anterior posterior direction but most particularly mouth opening. They may do this using the Mallampati test which is a grading of visibility of mouth structures with the patient sitting in a head neutral position; the patient is asked to open their mouth as wide as possible and fully protrude their tongue. If this gives full visibility of the tonsils, uvula and soft palate this is a good sign but if only the hard palate can be seen this is a sign that conventional intubation might be difficult.

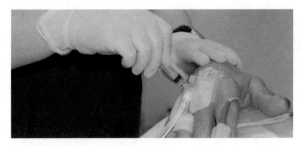

Anaesthesia is usually induced IV.

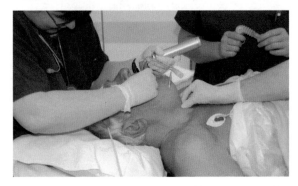

Intubation. The patient has been induced IV & the anaesthetic physician's assistant is passing an oral tube though the vocal cords into the trachea with direct vision using the laryngoscope. This is helped by an assistant putting downward pressure on the larynx.

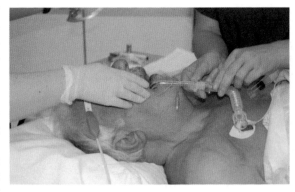

Once in place the tube is connected to the anaesthetic circuit and secured. The position is checked by inflating the lungs by squeezing the gas reservoir bag and listening to the chest with a stethoscope. The correct position will also be confirmed by looking at the observation monitor which will show the presence of expired CO_2. The eyes are taped shut and protected.

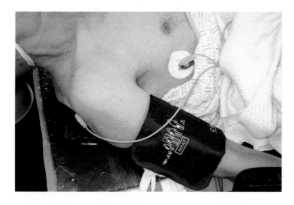

Everyone is monitored with ECG and blood pressure

If a patient is given a conventional anaesthetic induction with propofol and a muscle relaxant and then the anaesthetist cannot place a tube in the trachea this is potentially dangerous as the patient will not be able to breathe and the airway might be lost. An alternative technique is to give the patient a gas induction so that he breathes into a deep anaesthetic without a muscle relaxant. However this might be problematical if it is difficult to get a good air seal with a face mask because of abnormal anatomy, facial trauma or a beard, or if the patient is obese and might de-saturate their oxygen concentration quickly. In days of yore some anaesthetists practised the blind nasal intubation in which the patient was induced and then a tube was passed in through the nose and manipulated into the trachea without direct vision. The success of this was based on skill, experience, luck and bravado. This is considered to be too risky nowadays so for potentially difficult intubation cases the fibre optic intubation technique is used by an anaesthetist who has received special training and has a special interest and skill.

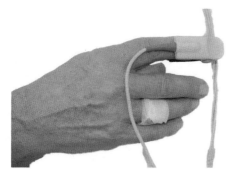

Pulse oximeter on forefinger. This monitors oxygen saturation and pulse rate. A decorative ring is taped.

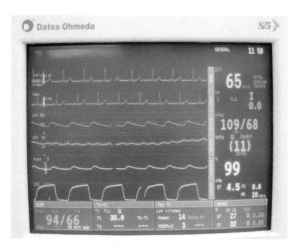

The video monitor during a major case. It shows ECG, pulse rate, blood pressure, O2 saturation, expired CO2, central venous pressure, direct arterial pressure & temperature.

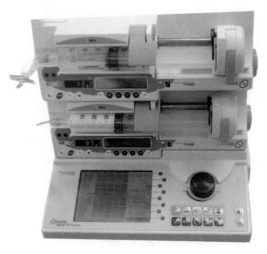

TIVA. Propofol and Remifentanil being administered by continuous infusion from a syringe driver.

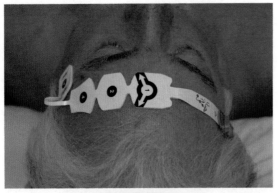

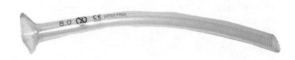

A nasal airway placed after the tube is removed to prevent airway obstruction during recovery.

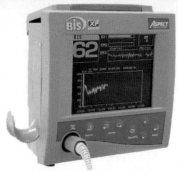

Bispectral index cerebral function monitor. It monitors the depth of anaesthesia by recording electrical activity (Electroencephalography or EEG).

<u>**Breathing circuit**</u>

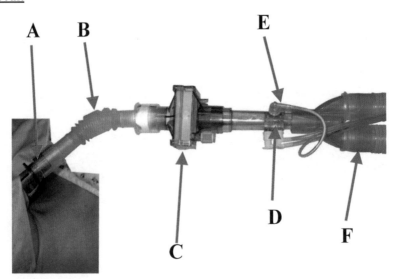

A: Endotrachael tube passing into patient's mouth B: Connector to tube C: Gas filter/humidifier D: Gas pressure/flow monitor E: Gas (O_2, N_2O and anaesthetic vapour monitor system F: Anaesthetic gases circuit, in and out

Anaesthetic machine

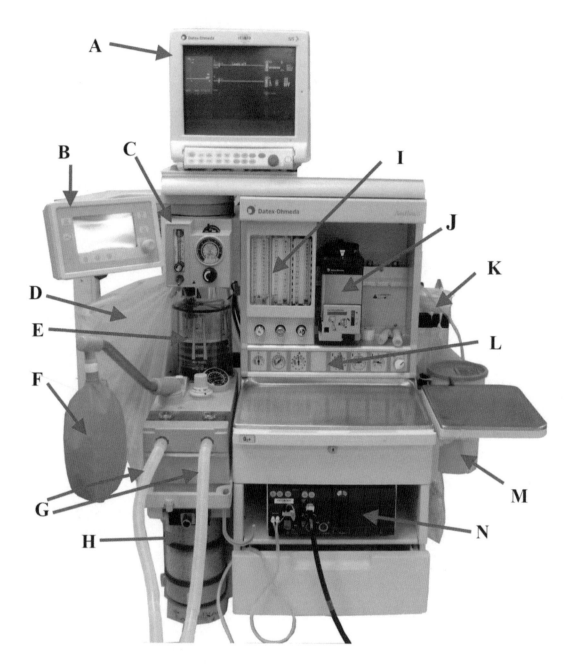

A: *Monitor* B: *Ventilator control system* C: *Suction control* D: *Clinical waste bag* E: *Ventilator bellows* F: *Reservoir bag* G: *Anaesthetic gas circuit, in and out* H: *C0₂ scavenger* I: *Gases flow meters* J: *Vaporiser for anaesthetic* K: *Suction chamber* L: *Gas pressure gauges* M: *Sharps box* N: *Monitoring modules for blood pressure, O₂ saturation, arterial pressure, central venous pressure, temperature*

Fibre optic intubation

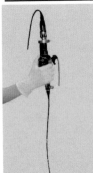

1. *A conventional endoscope is used. This has a fibre optic light source, a suction portal and fibres which allow vision through the end either directly or via a video display.*

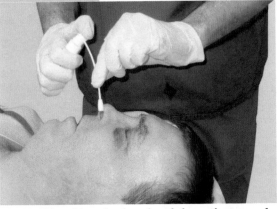

2. *An IV catheter is placed and the patient may be sedated with Remifentanil, a short acting opiate, and given some Glycopyrronium, an antimuscarinic to dry up nasal and salivary secretions. Topical local anaesthetic is placed in the nose.*

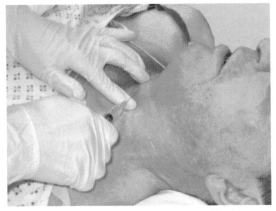

3. *Local anaesthetic is injected into the larynx to facilitate the passing of the tube through the vocal cords.*

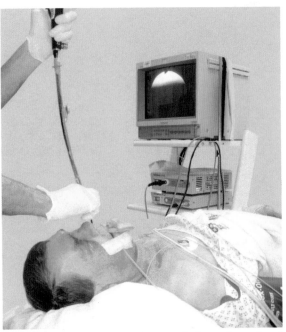

4. *The endoscope is passed through the endotrachael tube and is then advanced down to the larynx and through the vocal cords into the trachea, facilitated by vision though the scope displayed on the VDU.*

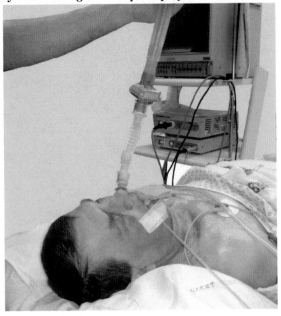

5. *Once the end of the endoscope has passed into the trachea the tube can be safely passed over it into the trachea. The scope is then removed and the tube can be attached to the anaesthetic breathing circuit.*

43. <u>Understanding Tracheostomy</u>

A tracheostomy, where a tube is inserted through the skin of the anterior neck directly into the trachea, is used routinely in OMFS to facilitate breathing or ventilation of the lungs. We use the technique principally in major cancer cases where the surgery itself, or bleeding or swelling afterwards, may potentially obstruct the airway. It thus makes the process safer and reduces risk. It will also facilitate providing a second anaesthetic in the post-operative period if something should go wrong, such as bleeding or flap failure. The second use in OMFS is following major facial trauma where there may be multiple fractures of the mandible, tongue swelling or fragments of broken tooth or bleeding which might compromise the airway.

There are other indications for tracheostomy, such as maintenance of the airway in patients who have reduced consciousness or who need longer term artificial ventilation of the lungs on an intensive care unit.

Tracheostomy has traditionally been the work of ENT surgeons and they usually provide a tracheostomy service for patients of other specialities in the hospital. In some hospitals OMF surgeons are involved with providing this service.

Tracheostomy is most commonly carried out during an open operation with a patient under general anaesthesia but in intensive care units it may be performed using a percutaneous technique by the intensive care physicians.

Following tracheostomy the two main concerns are that the tube might block or become displaced. The patient should therefore be looked after by nurses who are skilled in the monitoring of patients with tracheostomy and are skilled in their care. This usually means they are on an ENT or OMFS ward, a powerful argument for the two specialities to share facilities. Equipment should be available on the ward to deal with tracheostomy emergencies (blockage or displacement); it is often kept in a 'tracheostomy box' containing tracheostomy tubes, tracheal dilators, inner tubes, tapes etc. A nasendoscope is used in the diagnosis of a displaced tracheostomy tube.

Good care should reduce the risk of blockage or displacement. Patients should breathe air that has been humidified which will reduce the formation of thick

Tracheostomy

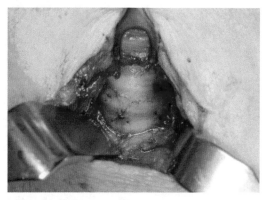

1. Under endo-tracheal anaesthesia patient is positioned with neck extended. Trachea is exposed thorough horizontal incision.

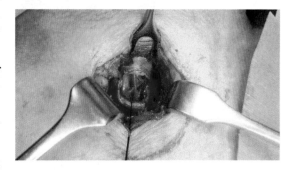

2. A window is cut in trachea at level of 2nd & 3rd tracheal ring. The anaesthetic tube is seen within.

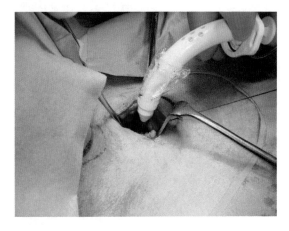

3. The anaesthetist withdraws the endotracheal tube as the tracheostomy tube is introduced.

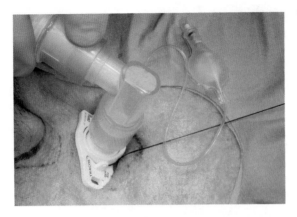

4. The anaesthetic circuit is attached to the tube, the cuff is inflated and the tube is secured to the patient with sutures and/or tape around the

tenacious sputum. Sputum accumulation can be reduced by regular suction through the tube using a thin (size 2) catheter tube inserted and slowly withdrawn. The inner tube should be removed by the nursing staff at regular intervals and washed or replaced. The tube should be securely fixed to the patient by sutures or tape around the neck; this should be checked regularly. The whole tracheostomy tube should be changed every 7 to 10 days. In most of our patients the tube will not be needed after a few days post-operation.

It is desirable that the tracheostomy be removed as soon as it is not needed. The air should be removed from the cuff and the tube should be suctioned to remove secretions which might have accumulated above the cuff. Before removing the tube it is essential that the patient is able to breathe around the tube which may be facilitated by using a fenestrated tube. The tube can be blocked off for a while so that we can be confident that the patient no longer needs it. The speech and language therapist can be consulted as they have expertise in airway patency. Tube removal is best carried out first thing on a week day morning ensuring there are sufficient trained staff available to deal with any problems.

Outer tracheostomy tube

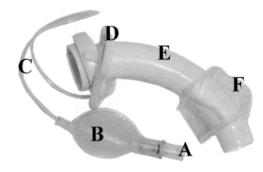

A: *Air introduction port* B: *Air reservoir (expands when cuff is inflated)* C: *Air connecting tube to cuff* D: *Flange* E: *Outer tube shaft* G: *Air cuff*

Introducer: *Is placed inside outer tube when tube is inserted into trachea at operation.*

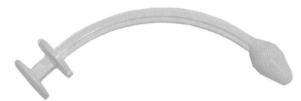

Inner tube: Locks in place in outer tube & can be removed for cleaning.

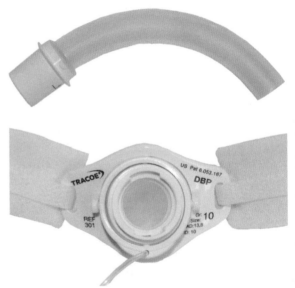

Outer tube from front: Shows flange marked with size, lock for inner tube, cuff air tube and neck attachment tape.

44. The Head & Neck Cancer Multidisciplinary Team (MDT)

It is important that trainees in any speciality of dentistry are able to see and understand the management of potentially malignant lesions in the mouth. There should be plenty of opportunity for you to do this within a department of OMFS but you will also get, and should seize, the opportunity to see and feel cancers as well as take histories from patients and observe their treatment; this will help develop your suspicion of unusual conditions you see in the mouth. When practising any form of clinical dentistry a familiarity with cancer can only help with recognition and early diagnosis.

OMFS as a speciality is heavily committed to patients with cancer and is ideally placed with medical, surgical and dental training to manage it. As a dentally qualified trainee you will probably be involved in taking biopsies and assisting at surgery, some of which can be quite lengthy. You should not be involved in making any decisions about patient treatment as you will not be trained or qualified to do so and this will include making any decisions about post-operative management on the ward. You may however be called by the nurses if a patient has an actual or perceived problem. You should always pass on the concern to someone more senior, usually the Specialist Registrar or Consultant. In well run departments post op cancer patients will be visited by a Consultant or Specialist Registrar at least daily until they are fit enough to go home and usually twice a day in the first few days.

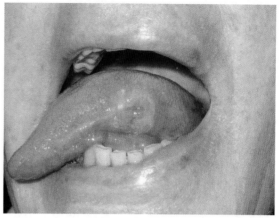

Infiltrating squamous cancer floor of the tongue. It was sore and starting to get painful. We do not yet know if we have cured it.

Mouth cancer will be managed, along with other cancers of the upper aero digestive tract, by the 'Head and Neck' Oncology Multidisciplinary Team (MDT). This will have core members who will include OMFS surgeons, ENT surgeons, clinical oncologists, radiologist, pathologist and a specialist head and neck oncology nurse; there may also be a plastic surgeon. There will usually be two of each type of surgeon and for each specialist there will be a deputy who will be available when someone is away so treatment will not be delayed. There will also be non-core members of the team who will consist of ward nurses, Macmillan nurses, who are specialists in cancer care out of the hospital, speech and language therapists who are specialists in problems of speech and swallowing, as well as dietician, physiotherapist, restorative dentist and dental hygienist.

The team will usually be based in a large hospital or hospitals close to the centre of the area they serve and should have a catchment of more than one million population. This will vary and may be less if there is a geographical reason for it to facilitate access to treatment in rural areas. In larger teams the core member may specialise completely in cancer but more usually they will have a major interest in it and will do some other non-cancer work as well.

The teams work to national agreed protocols and standards and intermittently will have accreditation visits to ensure that these standards are being met. The team should be collecting data on patient numbers, diagnosis, stage at presentation and mortality and morbidity data. It is now impossible for

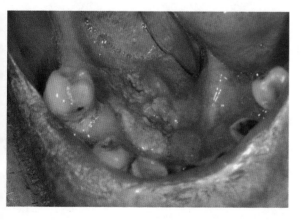

Squamous cancer floor of the mouth. Patient was alerted to it by pain; however when small the cancers will be painless. Patient was a heavy smoker and drinker of sprits; he also had an inoperable cancer of the oesophagus.

new surgeons to set themselves up carrying out cancer work in isolation without being part of a proper team.

The team activity will be based around a Multidisciplinary Team (MDT) meeting which will usually occur once a week. The exact format of the meeting will vary between hospitals but the principle will be that cases will be discussed and patients seen after diagnosis but before treatment, and again after surgery so that they have the opinion of at least two surgeons and an oncologist about the benefits and risks of available treatment. Colleagues can therefore support each other by offering their own special expertise and knowledge, by ensuring treatment continues when someone is away and ensuring that advances in treatment are assimilated into the team and patients are protected from eccentric management options. The team approach is particularly helpful when things don't go as planned.

Patients with suspected cancer of mouth, nasal passages, pharynx, larynx or thyroid or who present with a neck lump are usually referred to the OMFS or ENT departments who carry out the investigation, which will include a biopsy. Some patients come though neck lump clinics run by OMFS or ENT surgeons. After diagnosis they are brought to the MDT where recommendations for treatment are made. The politically correct way of deciding treatment is for the patient to decide following advice from the professional. In practice patients are generally bewildered by this and almost always want the team to make the decision and we are happy to make recommendations which they usually follow. The decisions are usually fairly easy to make as the

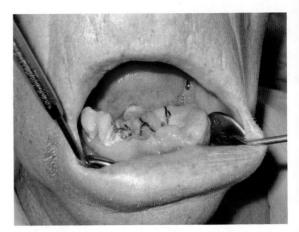

Large squamous carcinoma of the lower alveolus at presentation. The GP had treated it with mouthwashes and the dentist with antibiotics. When this didn't work he took the teeth out, hence the black silk sutures. By the time the patient was seen in hospital the tumour was deeply infiltrating into the mandible. While in hospital you must see as many cancers as possible so that you may recognise them, but any lesion you don't recognise must be treated with suspicion.

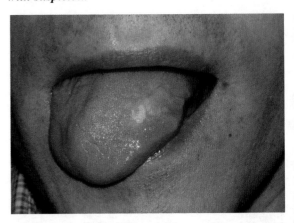

A happier tale. This patient had no symptoms & had not noticed the white patch on his tongue. His dentist referred him in. A biopsy showed severe epithelial dysplasia so the whole patch was removed with CO_2 laser. Within it the pathologist found a squamous cancer penetrating 0.7 mms. A wider local excision was carried out.

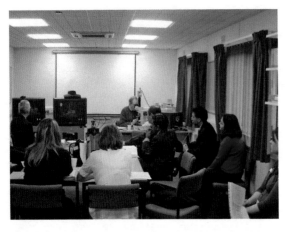

MDT meeting. The Pathologist is demonstrating the histology for the case under discussion.

presentation of the disease and pattern is very repetitive, especially where the patient comes with early disease which is amenable to treatment and where a cure can be attempted. This can be more difficult in the case where the disease is advanced at presentation and a cure is unlikely. In this case treatment to palliate the symptoms is more realistic.

Occasionally we get patients who are quite adamant that they do not want surgery when we recommend it but will submit to radiotherapy. Experience has shown us that they are sometimes right and radiotherapy is curative alone; this is because we are dealing with an unpredictable disease. Each individual tumour has its own (abnormal) genetic make-up and hence its own personality and some behave themselves when treated but others have decided at the outset they are going to be awkward and continue to grow whatever we throw at them. It is not unusual for cancers of the tongue, especially, to erupt around the margins of a surgical resection, even though the histopathology suggests an adequate surgical margin, and then to be only temporarily impeded by post-operative radiotherapy.

Most oral cancers are managed initially by surgery. Following diagnosis by biopsy the MDT will look at the slides of the tumour with the Pathologist and scans of head and neck, as well as the chest, with a radiologist; a recommendation for treatment will be made. Following surgery the patient will attend the MDT clinic again and the team will look at the specimen with the pathologist and, depending upon the width of the resection margins, presence or otherwise of lymph node involvement, peri-neural or vascular invasion, a recommendation may be made to have post-operative radiotherapy or chemotherapy; this should start within six weeks of surgery. Radiotherapy is usually provided daily over a period of about six weeks. Chemotherapy may be given at the same time as radiotherapy. Usually the patients are followed up once a month for the first year, two monthly for the second year and then three monthly for another and then twice in the fourth year. They are then discharged at five years. Most of our patients have squamous cell carcinoma. If they are going to get recurrent disease this usually is apparent with the first year after

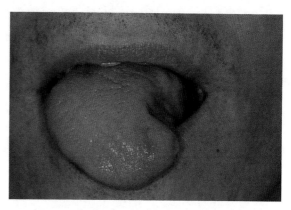

The cancer was caught early and four years later the residual tongue deformity caused no morbidity.

diagnosis. Most remaining failures manifest themselves between one and two years and it is unusual for patients to get recurrent disease after two years. Of course patients who have had head and neck cancer are at increased risk of getting a second primary, particularly if they continue to smoke. The more unusual tumour may behave differently; for example some muco-epidermoid cancers can behave very well and adenocystic cancers have a nearly 100% five year survival rate but tend to recur much later so that the 15 year survival is low. Oro-pharyngeal squamous cancers related to human papilloma virus infection tend to occur in younger patients and have an overall better prognosis than other squamous carcinomas of the oral cavity.

Key Points

- OMFS - part of the multidisciplinary team - treating head and neck cancer including mouth cancer
- Junior trainees are involved in taking biopsies, dental assessment and assisting in surgery
- Daily ward round by Specialist Registrar and sometimes Consultants
- Head and Neck Oncology Multidisciplinary Team (MDT) consists of surgeons, clinical oncologists, radiologists, pathologists, clinical nurse specialist, speech & language therapists, restorative dentists and dental hygienist, physiotherapist, dieticians.

- Weekly MDT conference to discuss treatment plan before and after treatment including surgery
- The MDT work to national agreed protocol and standards, and collect data for audit and clinical governance
- Staging mouth cancer – size of proven cancer, nodal involvement by MRI scan of head and neck, and possible metastasis by CT chest
- Following surgery, MDT discussion based on specimen's resection margins, lymph node involvement, perineural or vascular invasion may suggest adjuvant radiotherapy or chemo-radiotherapy
- Follow up usually monthly for the first year with widening gaps and discharge after 5 years

45. <u>Understanding a Major Cancer Case</u>

The management of patients with malignant disease is different in many respects from our other work. Chiefly the patients tend to be more elderly, their condition is life threatening, and they are more likely to have co-existing systemic disease; they are more likely to suffer complications of their treatment. In addition, their surgery is usually more complicated. We will therefore present a short explanation of surgical management of a typical patient with a mouth cancer requiring ablative surgery and reconstruction.

First however we will clarify your role as a dental trainee in the management of such a patient. We believe it will be valuable for you to see a few of these cases and to know the history of the presentation and be familiar with the symptoms that the patient first experienced and in particular to examine the tumours so that you may have a heightened awareness of mouth cancer during your future career. However we would hope that you are not tempted to make any decisions or change the management of any patient without consulting your senior. You should always ask either the Specialist Registrar or Consultant if there is any doubt about a patient. In effect you will be observing the management of the patient, learning, possibly passing messages and assisting in some part where asked.

In most cases cancer of the mouth will be managed by surgery initially and may be followed by radiotherapy and possibly chemotherapy. In practical terms most of our patients will receive both surgery and radiotherapy.

Following diagnosis by biopsy the patient will have a thorough examination not only of the mouth but the neck for possible evidence of lymph node metastasis. This examination will include a full examination of the whole of the upper aero digestive tract with a fibre optic endoscope, as a patient with oral cancer has a chance of having a secondary primary metachronous cancer and clearly at present this will need treating.

The examination will include an OPG and assessment of the dentition. If the patient is likely to have radiotherapy then any suspect teeth in the line of treatment will need removing to reduce the risk of osteo-radionecrosis of the mandible which is a terrible affliction in its own right and must be avoided at all costs.

Part of the pre-operative assessment will include scanning, either CT or MRI scan or both. If the tumour is in the maxilla, or elsewhere is extensive, then a CT scan will be requested to demonstrate the extent of bone invasion. A CT of the chest is mandatory to exclude metastatic disease in the chest.

A main concern about all cancers will be the spread to the lymphatic drainage of the neck. An MRI scan can be helpful in diagnosis of cancerous infiltration of neck nodes. If enlarged or suspicious nodes are identified by palpation or on the scan then an ultrasound guided fine needle aspirate can be examined by a cytologist to determine whether there are metastatic cells present. An MRI will also help to delineate the degree of soft tissue invasion, particularly helpful in base of tongue tumours.

Pre-operative tests will usually include a full blood count to check the pre-operative haemoglobin level. This will be needed as a base line as we will be expecting a possibly significant blood loss. A cross match and request for about four units of blood is made to replace the red cells lost during surgery. Blood chemistry (urea and electrolytes), although not considered routine for most surgery, will be needed as we need to know the base line levels particularly of the potassium which will increase after a blood transfusion. Liver function tests are also not necessary for most routine surgery but will be needed for most head and neck cases. We will need to know if there are any metabolic consequences of metastatic disease (unusual) or of alcohol which is more common in oral malignancy. A large alcohol intake is a major risk factor for the disease. The liver function test will include albumin and globulins. A low protein level may result from a poor nutritional intake consequent upon the disease itself or from an alcohol diet. An ECG is usual because our patients are mostly elderly and may have existing or past cardiac disease.

Most patients with intra oral cancer will receive a neck dissection. Cancers in the tongue or anywhere in the floor of the mouth, especially large ones, have a good chance of already producing metastatic disease in the lymph nodes of the neck. This may be of an extent that it cannot be detected by clinical examination or scanning and so nodes must be examined microscopically. Lymphatic spread tends to occur

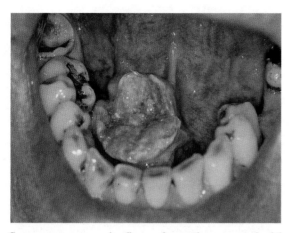

Squamous cancer in floor of mouth presented with pain. It is not involving the mandible. The treatment plan recommended to the patient by the head and neck oncology multidisciplinary team was a modified neck dissection, resection of the tumour and reconstruction with a free flap of skin and fascia taken from the forearm (radial forearm flap). This is the standard operation used in this situation. The mandible was not invaded so bone was not resected. The surgery was followed by radiotherapy. The bad teeth in the line of the radiation were removed at operation.

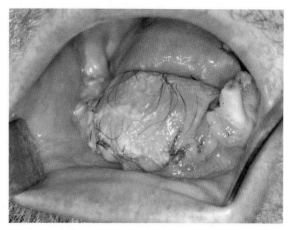

Three weeks later the radial forearm flap had taken nicely and was growing hair. The Vicryl sutures had not all dissolved yet. Radiotherapy was planned to start within six weeks; it stops the hair growth. At the time of writing six years had passed and the patient was alive and well .

sequentially from above downwards but in the case of lesions on the side of the tongue there may be skip lesions with lower nodes containing tumour while those above do not.

The radical neck dissection was described by Crile in 1904. It is the easiest neck dissection to perform and involves removal of most of the structures. It is still the operation of choice for advanced neck disease where there are several large nodes which suggest that spread outside the capsule of the node is likely. It involves removing all the structures in the neck superficial to the pre-vertebral fascia from the trapezius muscle behind to the midline of the neck anteriorly and from the clavicle inferiorly to the submandibular triangle superiorly. In addition to the nodes the sternomastoid muscle, the omohyoid muscle, the internal jugular vein, the submandibular salivary gland and the accessory nerve in the posterior triangle of the neck are removed.

The following structures must be preserved. The carotid artery: torrential haemorrhage will occur if damaged and if divided there will be very high incidence of stroke. The vagus nerve: heart rate will

increase and the recurrent laryngeal innovation to the vocal cords will be lost so that the patient would not be able to abduct the cord and would therefore have a hoarse voice. The hypoglossal nerve: if damaged there would be no tongue movement. This of course is not important if the resection includes hemi-glossectomy. In addition, by straying outside the proposed operation field it is possible to damage the phrenic nerve which lies just behind the pre-vertebral fascia. In this event the diaphragm on the affected side would move upward, decreasing the thoracic space for the lung and producing an increased risk of chest infection and atelectasis. Superiorly it is possible to damage the facial nerve which will lead to drooping of the face. On the left side of the neck the surgeon must keep a lookout for chyle draining from the thoracic duct. If seen it should be repaired; it will be quite difficult to see the duct itself.

However, more frequently we use a selective neck dissection which is permissible if there are one or two nodes without disease spread beyond their capsule. If neck disease is found to be more extensive than anticipated then a selective neck dissection may be converted into a radical one. The advantage of the selective neck dissection is twofold. Firstly it preserves the accessory nerve in the posterior triangle; the sacrifice of this nerve in most cases produces what is known as a shoulder syndrome due to the loss of its innovation to the trapezius muscle. The patient's shoulder droops; they are unable to lift their arm above their head and attempting to do so causes the scapula to wing out. Eventually the shoulder becomes painful which can be helped to a certain extent by aggressive physiotherapy but it is sacrifice of this nerve that causes the major morbidity following a radical neck dissection.

The selective neck dissection relies on the fact that oral tumours, particularly anterior ones, are unlikely to spread to the nodes of the posterior triangle. If any nodes, or suspicion thereof, are found in the posterior triangle at operation the nerve must be sacrificed because preservation of it is not an oncologically sound procedure. The selective neck dissection also conserves the internal jugular vein; dissection of the nodes from around the vein makes the procedure fiddly and more prolonged. There are two reasons to preserve this vein. Firstly if there is disease in both sides of the neck sacrificing both veins will mean that the only drainage from the head will be through the vertebral veins. This will lead to severe swelling of the head although this will probably settle with time. The most usual reason for preserving the internal jugular vein is to allow anastomosis of the venous drainage from the free flap used to reconstruct the defect caused by the cancer ablation surgery.

For a patient with a small primary tumour with no evidence of neck disease the clinician will have to decide whether to closely observe the neck over a period of time for evidence neck metastases or carry out a selective neck dissection with removal of the primary tumour, knowing that many patients will have surgery in which no cancer is detected on subsequent histological examination. A third method which is under investigation is biopsy of the sentinel node in the neck. This is the first node to receive lymphatic drainage from the tumour area. It is identified with nuclear medicine imaging by injecting the patient the day before with technetium labelled colloid which gives off gamma rays. The node is removed via a small neck incision at the time of removal of the primary tumour and subjected to extensive histological examination. If micro-metastases are found a selective neck dissection is carried out within a couple of weeks.

Following a radical or selective neck dissection a specimen will be subjected to histology. Presence of disease in one node if cleanly removed will not adversely affect the prognosis, and radiotherapy may not be needed. However if there are more nodes than this affected then post-operative radiotherapy will be indicated, and spread through the capsule of the lymph node would have severely compromised the prognosis for a cure. Chemo-radiotherapy may also be offered to patients with good general health.

We will now return to the subject of pre-operative preparation and in particular to the preparation for feeding the patient after the operation. You will understand that if we are resecting a tumour in the oral cavity and at the same time dissecting the neck nodes there will be direct communication between the mouth and neck giving direct access for saliva, food and drink into the tissues of the neck. The floor of the mouth will be reconstructed at the time of operation, in most cases by a radial forearm free flap. The radial forearm flap is delicate and any breakdown of the suture line at the edge of the wound will encourage a litre and a half of saliva and anything else swallowed to drain in the neck and eventually out through the most inferior neck wound which will break down. This complication is known as an oro-cutaneous or salivary fistula and although it usually dries up with time this may take two or three months and in the meantime sepsis in the neck will compromise the pedicle and anastomosis of the free flap which may die as a result.

In order to minimize the risk of this disastrous complication we stop the patient taking anything by mouth for several post-operative days. During this time the patient must be fed through a tube passing directly into the stomach and thus by-passing the mouth. This is usually achieved with a fine bore tube passed through the abdominal skin by a radiologist using ultrasound as PUG (percutaneous ultrasound guided gastrostomy) or RIG (radiologically inserted gastrostomy). This gastrostomy tube is placed a few days before the patient is admitted to the hospital for surgery. They are trained to use the tube themselves as this can be kept in place for months and may be useful later if they are to have radiotherapy which causes severe mucosal inflammation and hence pain during swallowing so that supplemental feeding through a tube is desirable.

Once all investigations have been completed, blood has been ordered, a gastrostomy tube fitted and the patient has been through the consenting process with the Consultant, the patient is admitted to the hospital for the operation, usually the night before, after which they are kept 'nil by mouth'.

In theatre the patient is anaesthetized in the anaesthetic induction room but there are several things to be done before the resection starts. Firstly the anaesthetist will secure intravenous access for giving fluids, drugs and blood. A central line will be passed from probably the femoral or subclavian veins up into the right atrium; occasionally the internal jugular vein will be used. This is to measure central venous pressure so that the anaesthetist can accurately decide how much fluid must be given to replace that which has been lost. An arterial line will be placed usually into a radial artery; this will be used to accurately monitor blood pressure during the procedure and will be much more accurate for rapid changes of blood pressure, for example after a sudden blood loss, than a sphygmomanometer. The arterial line will be used to take samples of blood for estimation of blood gases if necessary, and the haemoglobin. A pulse oximeter will be placed on the finger to read the pulse rate and oxygen saturation.

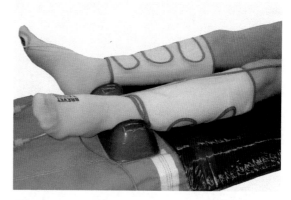

The patient on the operating table. He wears thrombo embolic deterrent (TED) stockings, placed on him on the ward with further compression to the calves placed in theatre. His ankles rest on soft gel pads and he lies on a soft warming pad.

After all the lines have been placed, which with the anaesthetic may take up to an hour, the patient is moved to the theatre where a urinary catheter is placed. This allows the urinary outflow to be measured (this will be decreased if inadequate fluid is replaced). The catheter will contain a temperature probe to measure core temperature (decreased if the patient is shocked).

The patient will be placed on a warming pad through which warm fluid will be pumped to maintain body temperature as the operation will be long, and compression stockings will be placed on the legs to gently compress the calves throughout the operation, discouraging the formation of thrombus in the deep veins of the legs. A thrombosis of the deep veins can be disastrous; it might cause venous ulceration of the leg and if a portion of clot should detach and form an embolus in the lungs it can cause sudden death. A fine bore naso gastric tube will probably be placed so that gastric secretions can be aspirated during the operation.

The operative procedure usually starts with a tracheostomy. A cuffed tracheostomy tube is placed. This removes the inconvenience of having to operate around a nasal or oral tube which may interfere with the surgery but more importantly it makes the whole post-operative period safer, as the airway will not be compromised by swelling or bleeding, and, in the unlikely event that the patient has to return to theatre for attention to bleeding or the flap re-anaesthetizing, will be a much simpler and safer procedure. The tracheostomy tube is usually removed three or four days post op when we are confident that the patient

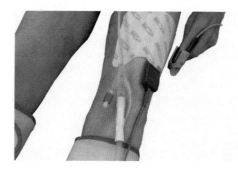

On his leg is a diathermy pad; on his finger a pulse oximeter. The urinary catheter is shown. It has three ports: one is to blow up the retaining balloon in the bladder with water, another is to drain the urine, which is measured. The third is the temperature probe.

can breathe through their mouth or nose and that there are no complications making re-anaesthetizing likely.

Following tracheostomy the patient is prepared (prepped) with the skin wiped with disinfectant solution, usually Povidone iodine or Savlon, and draped with sterile surgical drapes. The operation proper can begin. The surgery starts with the neck dissection and then usually proceeds to resection of the primary tumour. The aim is to remove all the lymph nodes without breaching the capsules of the glands and the primary tumour with a good surgical margin (usually 1 - 2 cms). After the resection the specimen is removed and placed on a cork board and pinned out so that it can be orientated by the pathologist who will need to dissect the specimen. He will need to know which bit he is dealing with so that he is able to produce an accurate report for staging purposes. Further samples may be taken from the margins of the 'clean' resection wound and sent for histology in separate bottles for frozen sections during surgery. This is useful as an additional check as the specimen will shrink and the pathologist's reported clearance margin may not be accurate so it will be helpful for reassurance that the tumour has been cleared (or otherwise) which will contribute to the decision on whether radiotherapy is recommended.

Following resection reconstruction is carried out, typically with a radial forearm flap, which is usually plumbed into the lingual or facial artery and internal jugular vein. Raising the flap from the forearm can be started by another maxillofacial surgeon while the resection is being completed.

Following surgery the patient will go back to the ward. It will need to be a ward which is used to looking after patients with tracheostomy. The patient may be admitted to an Intensive Care Unit if they are medically unfit before surgery; often this is because of ischaemic heart or respiratory disease. If this is the case they may be sedated and respiratory ventilation taken over by machine or the patient may breathe spontaneously assisted by CPAP (continuous positive airways pressure) or PEEP (positive end expiratory pressure). These improve airways expansion and respiratory exchange and decrease the risk of atelectasis (peripheral airway collapse).

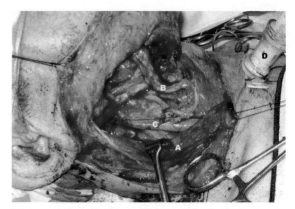

The neck completed before closing. A is the sternomastoid muscle held back by a retractor. B is the pedicle running up to the flap in the floor of the mouth. C is the internal jugular vein with the pedicle vein attached to its side. D is the tracheostomy tube.

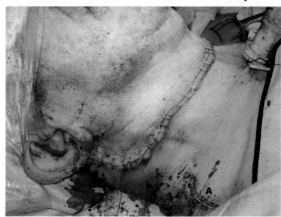

Neck closed with staples. They are quick to put in and clean and easy to remove 10 days later. This incision gives a very acceptable cosmetic result. A is a suction drain to prevent haematoma formation.

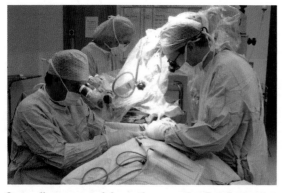

Once disconnected from the arm the flap is put into place and the radial artery is anastomosed to the lingual or facial artery and the veins to the internal jugular. The surgeon is using an operating microscope as the arteries are 1 mm diameter but the assistant is using operating loupes. This is micro-vascular surgery.

Once back on the ward post-operative medication will need to be reviewed and prescribed. This will now include subcutaneous enoxaparin given to prevent deep vein thrombosis. The patient should also have TED (thrombo embolic deterrent) stockings for the same purpose. Enteral feeding will be started through the gastrostomy tube; the feed will be prescribed by a dietician. The patient should now be getting all their fluids via the tube, and the intravenous drip may be discontinued but the cannula should be retained for access of medication, for example antibiotics.

On the first post-operative day the patient will remain in bed but by the second day they should be encouraged to sit out of bed for a few hours in the

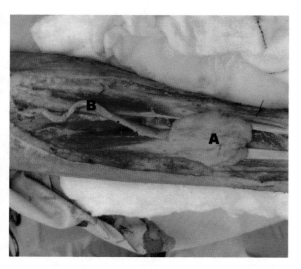

The radial forearm flap raised but not yet disconnected from the arm. It consists of skin and fascia (fascio-cutaneous). The flap A which is used to reconstruct the floor of the mouth is attached by the pedicle which consists of the radial artery and the small veins which accompany it (vena comitans). The hand is kept vital by blood supply from the ulnar artery. C is the wrist. If the mandible is to be resected a compound flap can be raised with the radius used to reconstruct the bone defect, but more commonly we use a free flap from the iliac crest or fibula from the leg.

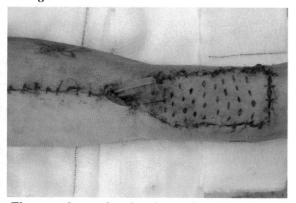

The arm donor site closed, usually with a V to Y advancement of skin, but in this case a skin graft has been used. A drain is placed to allow seepage of any bleeding. It is then bandaged.

morning or afternoon. They should have their haemoglobin and blood chemistry retested on the second morning. Haemoglobin should ideally be about 10 for the best chance of flap survival. The tracheostomy should be given regular suction and humidification to prevent crusting in the tube. The suction drains should be reviewed regularly. The nurses should have recorded the amount of drainage and those draining little or nothing should be removed by day three, retaining perhaps one drain at the bottom of the neck.

The urinary catheter will have been placed to monitor the urinary output during the operation and for the first 24 hours. The nurses usually appreciate its being retained for the purpose of convenience until the patient is mobilized. This should be permissible for another two or three days but thereafter it should be removed and the patient should be encouraged to go to the bathroom or otherwise use a bottle. Prolonged retention of the catheter will pre-dispose to urinary tract infection or ulceration and possibly stenosis of the urethra. It is a good policy to order the removal of one or two lines or tubes each morning on the ward round. The patient can then see this as a positive progression towards normality over the next few days.

It is important that the patient should have adequate pain relief. This is best achieved with an intravenous catheter attached to a syringe in a pump containing morphine which is dispensed regularly, with an additional amount being given by the patient pressing a button if they are in pain (this is called PCA or patient controlled analgesia). These do not tend to be very painful operations and the PCA will rarely be required after a couple of days when regular paracetamol given through the gastrostomy tube and supplemented by opioid analgesics prescribed on an 'as required' basis will be more appropriate.

A frequent problem in the post-operative period is with sleeping. We have found that a low dose of one of the more sedating tricyclic antidepressants such as dothiepin in the evening may help with this as well as having a beneficial effect on the mood later on. Usually in the first day or two after the operation the patients are in a very positive mood, even sometimes euphoric having discovered that they have got through the dreaded operation. They do however tend to get fed up by the end of the first week when they are getting stronger and are disconnected from all the lines and tubes except for the enteral feeding and are hanging around in hospital waiting for their flap to heal sufficiently for them to eat.

At about day three or four the tracheostomy tube should be removed. The cuff in the tube should have been let down on day two and now, by placing a gloved finger over the orifice of the tube, it is possible to see if the patient can breathe round it and through the nose or mouth. If so the tube can be removed and a dressing placed over the wound which usually heals spontaneously. If after a few days the tracheostomy continues to blow it should be sutured on the ward with local anaesthetic.

At a varying time, depending on the circumstances or local policy which in our case is seven days, the margins of the reconstruction in the mouth are inspected and if all is healing well the patient is allowed to take their first sips of water. If inspection the following morning reveals no problem with the wound margin the patient can progress to a sloppy diet and the following day to firmer things and be discharged home. Once they are able to take things by mouth enteral feeding is suspended but the PUG tube is retained in case it is needed during radiotherapy later.

Intra oral wounds are usually sutured with an absorbable suture such as Vicryl which does not need removing. Facial wounds are usually sutured with nylon and these are removed at six or seven days post-operatively. Neck wounds are usually closed with metal clips and these are removed alternately at nine or ten days.

We will conclude with a few words about relatives. Occasionally they will turn up in the evening or at the weekend and want to speak to the doctor and the nurse will call you. We would strongly advise you avoid discussion as you will not be in a position to provide a detailed explanation and information that they want to know about prognosis and you should always suggest that they see the Consultant in charge of the case during normal working hours. Our experience has been that less experienced clinicians tend to give too optimistic an outlook based on experience of too few cases.

Key Points

• After biopsy confirmation of mouth cancer – flexible nasendoscopy to examine upper aero-digestive tract for metachronous cancer

• OPG and dental assessment for removal of unrestorable dentition during surgery to avoid osteoradionecrosis of mandible

• MRI of head and neck, CT maxilla and mandible is bone invasion is suspected, CT chest for lung metastases

• Blood tests – FBC, Cross match 6 units of blood, Us & Es, LFT and clotting screen

• Neck dissection for staging the neck in small cancer and advanced neck disease

• Radical neck dissection for advanced neck disease

• Selective neck dissection for early neck disease or staging the neck for micrometases

• Defect after major cancer resection requires tissue reconstruction – e.g. radial forearm free flap (RFFF) for soft tissue reconstruction

• On Induction by anaesthetist – iv access, central line, arterial line, pulse oximeter, urinary catheterisation, temperature probe insertion, warming blanket, thrombo-embolic deterrant (TED) stockings with calves compression device, diathermy pad on thigh

• Tracheostomy, neck dissection, resection of primary tumour, pinning out the specimen, frozen section for clean surgical margins, reconstruction

• High dependency or intensive care bed usually required for first 24 hours

• Postoperative care – regular flap monitoring according to local protocol, 'nil by mouth' and nasogastric or gastrostomy tube feed for a week; subcutaneous anticoagulants, TED stocking, regular suction and humidifaction of tracheostomy tube, blood tests, pain relief using patient-controlled analgesia

46. <u>Understanding Radiotherapy and its Oral Complications</u>

Oral cancer is primarily squamous cell which is generally sensitive to radiotherapy. Radiotherapy uses high energy ionizing radiation to generate free radicals which break double-stranded DNA thus damaging the reproductive activity of cells leading to their death when they attempt to divide at mitosis; they are then removed by the body's own defence mechanism. Normal cells are damaged in the same way as malignant cells but unlike the cancer cells they have the ability to repair; they are thus much less affected.

Mouth cancer is usually treated primarily by surgery with radiotherapy used as an adjunct, normally afterwards. The blood supply of the normal tissues is adversely affected by radiotherapy and thus reduces their ability to heal which is why surgery is usually done first. Early cancers are often treated with surgery alone. The indications for radiotherapy include positive lymph nodes in the neck, particularly multiple nodes or spread outside the capsule of the glands, and close surgical margins or poor differentiation of the tumour as seen in the histology of the surgical specimens.

Oro-pharyngeal cancer (base of tongue, tonsil and pharynx) related to Human Papilloma Virus tends to occur in younger patients who tend to be to otherwise healthier with their condition unrelated to smoking and high alcohol. These cases usually have a better prognosis and are often treated using chemo-radiotherapy without surgery (more about this later).

Radiotherapy can be used as part of attempted 'curative' treatment to destroy the tumour or reduce the chance of it recurring after surgery or as part of 'palliative' treatment where the chance of a cure has passed and the clinician has the more limited expectation of shrinking the tumour or alleviating pain.

Brachytherapy is the term used where a radiation source is implanted in the patient. This was occasionally used in the head and neck, particularly for tongue cancers, but nowadays head and neck tumours are treated with external beam radiotherapy

<u>*Radiotherapy terminology*</u>

Curative: to cure the cancer
Adjuvant: after surgery to prevent recurrence
Neoadjuvant: to reduce the size of the tumour
prior to surgery
Palliative: to decrease severity and delay
progression

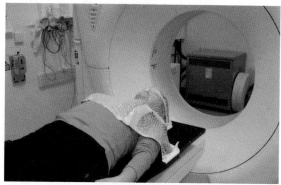

The patient is wearing a bespoke immobilization mask made of a thermoplastic material to hold her head in a reproducible position for a pre-treatment CT scan for radiotherapy planning.

delivered by a linear accelerator. Radiotherapy doses are expressed in Grays (Gy); a Gray is the radiation dose producing one joule of energy absorbed per kilogram of tissue. The dose is normally given divided into daily 'fractions' with time between which allows the normal tissues to recover; this helps maintain oxygenation of the tumour, hypoxic tissues being less sensitive to radiation. Once a radiotherapy regime has started it should not be interrupted. Delay in starting the radiotherapy is undesirable but it is not as detrimental to the outcome as interruption once treatment has started.

Three Dimensional Conformal Radiotherapy involves planning the treatment so that the radiotherapy is delivered to the tumour from different directions to maximize the dose to the tumour and reduce radiation to the normal surrounding tissues. The more sophisticated Intensity Modulated RadioTherapy (IMRT) is a refinement of Three Dimensional Conformal Radiotherapy. It involves many hundreds of small beams of radiation delivered to the tumour more precisely with improved sparing of the normal tissues. It is particularly used for head and neck cancer treatment where there are many structures which will benefit from avoiding radiation, such as the salivary glands, spinal cord and larynx. IMRT has been proved to reduce less long term side effects, particularly the salivary glands reducing xerostomia; radical IMRT is the standard of care that should be provided for head and neck cancer patients.

The planning process for radiotherapy treatment involves a CT scan taken with the patient wearing an

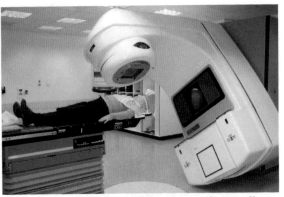

Patient receiving radiotherapy from linear accelerator wearing the mask to keep her head in reproducible position. (Simulated not a real patient)

immobilisation shell; the radiotherapist will then outline the tumour and sensitive structures e.g. spinal cord and salivary glands on the scan. An MRI scan can be overlaid onto the CT image on the computer to give more information but the actual doses will be calculated by the computer based on the density of the tumour which is informed by the CT scan. The radiotherapist then checks with the MRI scan that all the tumour has been included in the radiation fields. Three dimensional images can be very helpful in the planning. When the radiotherapist has prescribed the dose of radiation, marked out the volume to be treated and the structures to be avoided, a technologist plans the treatment on the computer.

The treatment is delivered from a linear accelerator radiotherapy machine with the patient immobilised with head and neck stabilisers and face masks. The radiographers who run the linear accelerator machines will go through a process of 'verification' to ensure that the plan that has been designed is being delivered. This is done with 'portal images' which are pictures of the exit radiation dose which are compared to what the planning computer says it should look like.

The most immediate side effect of radiotherapy to the head and neck is mucositis which usually manifests by the second or third week of treatment. It consists of widespread erythema, ulceration bleeding and pain. The oral and pharyngeal mucosa will become inflamed, sore and possibly ulcerated. Maintenance of oral hygiene will be difficult when the mouth is so sore and this may be helped by chlorhexidine mouthwash to help with plaque control. The discomfort will significantly affect the ability to chew and swallow and hence impede nutrition. This may to some extent be helped by using a high calorie liquid diet and topical analgesic mouthwash, gargle or spray (benzydamine hydrochloride). In many cases, particularly where radiotherapy is combined with chemotherapy, feeding is delivered through a gastrostomy tube placed before radiotherapy. A fine bore tube is inserted through the skin directly into the stomach, usually guided into the correct place with the aid of X-rays or ultrasound. In the longer term a gastrostomy often delays the patient's ability to swallow normally after the mucositis has settled; recovery may not be complete. The pain should therefore be treated and the patient encouraged to swallow something rather than rely entirely on the gastrostomy tube.

The cells of the mucosa exhibit a high rate of turnover so the mucositis can be expected to recover about three weeks after completion of treatment. However radiotherapy will have a permanent effect on the salivary glands, both major and minor, causing permanent damage and dryness of the mouth with such saliva as there is being thick. Whereas the effect is likely to be less with Intensity Modulated Radiotherapy the xerostomia caused will be permanent.

There are a variety of different saliva substitutes available to help with symptoms but our experience has been that patients often feel more comfortable carrying a bottle of water to use for symptomatic relief. Eventually patients seem to accommodate to the permanent dryness of the mouth with modulation of their diet but the xerostomia has a permanent effect on their dental health due to the decreased salivary buffering and a higher rate of caries will ensue; this may be helped with fluoride mouth rinses.

In the short term the mouth may be affected by secondary infection, particularly candidiasis, mucositis and ulceration. This may be helped by meticulous oral hygiene and antifungals such as miconazole or fluconazole. Herpes simplex may be reactivated which can be helped with acyclovir.

Probably the most serious complication of head and neck radiotherapy results from the effect of radiation on bone, particularly the mandible. The effect of the radiation is to obliterate blood vessels supplying the bone so that it is deprived of nutriments and oxygen. This severely curtails its capacity to remodel, resist infection and heal after trauma.

The resultant osteoradionecrosis may not be a problem to the patient until the bone is infected (particularly from periodontal or apical dental infection) or traumatised (particularly by dental extraction). Once infected the necrotic bone will drain pus into the mouth, become permanently exposed to the mouth and never heal. There will be permanent discharge with discomfort and unpleasant smell. There are likely to be acute exacerbations of the chronic infection with swelling and pain and a risk of pathological fracture. For very early osteoradionecrosis an attempt may be made to treat it with pentoxyphyzine, calcium and vitamin D; hyperbaric oxygen has been used but this modality seems to have fallen out of favour. If established there is a choice between leaving it and accepting the discomfort and disability or major surgery to remove all the necrotic bone and reconstruct with free vascularised bone grafts. Many of the patients will be elderly and frail and may not wish to have more major surgery after their cancer treatment. The damage to bone from radiotherapy is permanent so patients are at risk of septic osteoradionecrosis from dental infection or extraction for the remainder of their lives.

Radiotherapy will cause a similar reduction of vascularity to the soft tissues. This will cause reduced healing which is why we prefer to carry out surgery prior to radiotherapy. The skin may become pigmented and the soft tissues will also be prone to some degree of fibrosis which may be responsible for limitation of mouth opening, particularly if the medial pterygoid and masseter muscles are included in high dose volume of treatment.

In the long term radiotherapy increases the risk of the development of new tumours in the irradiated tissues. This has most significance in children who have received radiation for rare childhood tumours. It will also have a detrimental effect on growth in these children. Although it is clear that IMRT reduces the short term side effects of radiotherapy it does involve more of the normal tissues receiving radiation, although at a lower dose. It is possible that this may lead to a greater propensity to induce new tumours in the longer term although this is only speculation at the moment.

It is essential that all patients with oral, nasal or pharyngeal tumours should have a comprehensive assessment of their dentition as soon as they are diagnosed so that they are rendered dentally fit before treatment starts. In most centres the patients are assessed by a restorative dentist which will give the patient the opportunity to discuss future prosthetic rehabilitation. Any dental treatment or assessment should not be allowed to delay cancer treatment. We tend to take a pessimistic approach to future dental health and plan treatment accordingly. In assessing the dentition we acknowledge that most of the patients will be elderly and may have less than ideal periodontal conditions, that they may have less than ideal dental

health beforehand. Radiotherapy will cause xerostomia leading to greatly increased caries risk and that radiotherapy and surgery may lead to some degree of trismus making oral hygiene measures and dental inspection or treatment difficult. This and the experience that osteoradionecrosis is so miserable for the patient usually means we recommend a radical approach and that any teeth which are not completely healthy in terms of tooth substance and periodontium which are in the field of high dose radiation are removed before treatment.

Which Scan?

Computerized tomography (CT)

Most cases will have a CT scan. As it is based on X-rays it shows bone best. Radiotherapy is planned on a CT scan. Usually the scan is made after the patient is injected with a contrast medium to improve the image of the tumour. A CT of the chest is used to show up any metastatic tumour.

Magnetic Resonance Imaging (MRI)

Many cases of oral cancer can barely be seen on CT because the density of the tumour may be very close to that of the normal tissue. MRI will show up a huge signal variation so that soft tissue tumours can be seen clearly. Sometimes a CT is poor due to artifacts cause by dental fillings. All patients should therefore ideally have both scans especially for oral cancers.

Positron Emission Tomography (PET)

Is used when we don't know where the primary is. Sometimes a patient presents with metastatic nodes in the neck. If pan-endoscopy of the upper aerodigestive tract does not reveal the primary a PET scan may show up a suspicious area to be biopsied carefully.

PET scan shows inflammation so biopsies should be done after the scan as it might be difficult the differentiate inflammation from cancer. Often it will show up a tumour in the tongue base (with overlying mucosa looking intact) or in the pyriform fossa or tonsillar region that you haven't been able to get access to examine properly.

PET scans are useful for post treatment assessment in some cases particularly patients who have had chemo-radiotherapy for metastatic disease. A PET scan at three months post-treatment may show up residual disease which would indicate that neck dissection is required.

47. Understanding Chemotherapy and its Oral Complications

Chemotherapy is the use of anti-cancer drugs for the treatment of a wide variety of malignant conditions, particularly haemopoietic diseases such as leukaemias and lymphomas, but also for malignant cells metastasizing from solid tumours such as breast and bowel cancer. The agents used are usually given in combinations and at high dose to preferentially target actively dividing cancer cells. However they also have a wide range of nonspecific actions which will have an adverse effect on normal tissues, particularly those with a high rate of cell turnover. Thus the bone marrow, mucosa and salivary glands will be affected which will be detrimental to oral health and need consideration when patients need oral or dental surgery.

When used in the management of head and neck cancer chemotherapy is usually administered concomitantly with radiotherapy (chemoradiotherapy), usually for treatment of the more advanced cancers. For head and neck cancer cisplatin is used as a radiosensitizer together with cetuximab, an epidermal growth factor receptor blocker, which also acts as a radiosensitizer but with different toxicities to cisplatin. Chemotherapy is only very rarely used for head and neck cancer without radiotherapy; this may be for palliation when the chance of a cure has passed or occasionally used before radiotherapy to shrink the tumour down before radiotherapy starts.

Chemotherapy may cause mucositis leading to ulceration and discomfort with resulting difficulty in chewing and swallowing. Mucositis will be temporary and may be helped by mouthwashes such as benzydamine hydrochloride or ice. There will be taste dysfunction which will exacerbate the chewing and swallowing problems caused primarily by the mucositis; salivary gland function may be impaired by anti-cholinergic medication given as an adjunct to chemotherapy.

The most significant effect of chemotherapy affecting dental care will be myelosuppression (bone marrow suppression) causing leucopenia and thrombocytopenia. The reduced white cell count will lead to immunosuppression and, together with reduction in saliva production, will frequently lead to candidiasis which will further exacerbate the discomfort and dysphagia. Patients who are expected to be neutropenic as a result of chemotherapy are usually treated prophylactically with fluconazole; IV amphotericin may also be used.

Myelosuppression can be expected to be most problematical in patients receiving chemotherapy for leukaemias and lymphomas and most particularly those receiving stem cell transplants. Suppression will be significant for about six weeks after chemotherapy has finished and during this time the patient will be susceptible to becoming significantly unwell from dental infection or from other sources. An acute dental infection in a neutropenic patient may produce little or no pus (as there are few neutrophils from which pus can be formed) and hence may produce little or no pain but still cause the patient to be systemically unwell. A patient presenting with pyrexia during or soon after chemotherapy should be treated as an acute medical emergency and treated by the oncology team according to the hospital's 'neutropenic sepsis' policy.

Patients who are expected to become neutropenic from chemotherapy should ideally have their dentition optimised beforehand if time allows. An asymptomatic tooth with a chronic apical infection which has been draining, or a non-vital tooth with an apical radiolucency with no discharge may become dangerous during neutropenia when the balance of resistance will favour sepsis. Pre-treatment extraction is to be preferred.

Thrombocytopenia during or after chemotherapy may lead to bleeding from periodontal inflammation and prolonged bleeding following dental extraction. However we generally have far more platelets than are needed and the platelet count can be reduced quite considerably before bleeding becomes a practical problem. If an extraction is contemplated a haematologist should be consulted if the count is less than 50×10^9 per litre as they may prescribe a platelet transfusion but if the extraction is not urgent you can wait until it returns to above 100×10^9 per litre when the marrow is recovering from the chemotherapy.

Most of the side effects of chemotherapy on the mouth are temporary and will be expected to resolve with time.

48. <u>Understanding Diabetes and its Impact on Surgery</u>

With about 2.5 million diagnosed diabetics in the UK (10% type 1 & 90% type 2) plus, possibly, another half a million undiagnosed, it is inevitable that you will come across some who require OMFS surgery.

You will already know that diabetes mellitus is a chronic disease of carbohydrate, fat and protein metabolism. Type 1 diabetes is caused by the inability to produce insulin due to the autoimmune destruction of beta cells in the pancreas. Insulin is needed to facilitate the movement of glucose into cells from the blood stream. Type 1 diabetes usually presents in childhood; this can be quite sudden with a ketoacidosis attack. Type 1 diabetics require lifelong insulin replacement. Type 2 usually occurs in those over 40 years, but not necessarily. Most are obese and it can initially be asymptomatic. It results from resistance to insulin, decreased insulin secretion or excessive glucagon. Type 2 diabetics often do not need insulin replacement initially but many will eventually.

The best person to manage control of diabetes is the patient themselves, supervised by their general medical practitioner and his specialist diabetic nurse. In hospital as much control as possible should be vested in the patient themselves within local hospital protocol. For the patient who is hitherto undiagnosed or who has poor control or complications the specialist

---

Diabetic Treatment

Type 1

Typically by managing diet and exercise in conjunction with multiple injections of synthetic insulin monitored by blood glucose estimations. Often twice daily insulin with longer acting synthetic insulin. Sometimes short acting insulin before food. Some use subcutaneous insulin pump

Type 2

Diet, exercise, weight control
Metformin & Thiazolidinediones (glitazones) increase the effectiveness of insulin
Sulphonylureas increase insulin production by pancreas
Eventually will need insulin

---

diabetic team should take control; this will include a Consultant physician and a specialist nurse who will visit all in-patient diabetics daily. The anaesthetist will control the patient in the operative period. It is not the place of the surgeon to manage diabetes unguided by protocol or a specialist and certainly not the job of the dentally qualified trainee to change or initiate treatment. So this chapter is about understanding the process of good management.

Most type 1 diabetics originally present with one of the following symptoms: polyuria, polydipsia, weight loss, refractory visual problems (related to osmotic changes), muscle cramps and infections. Most type 2 diabetics present with polyuria, polydipsia, candidiasis and diabetic complications (see table). You should therefore bear in mind that the patient who comes with a large dental abscess may be one of the, perhaps, half a million previously undiagnosed diabetics who are immunocompromised by their condition. Patients with large abscesses should therefore have their glucose levels checked.

Surgery will affect diabetic glucose control by virtue of the patient being starved for anaesthesia or by being unable to eat normally as a result of the surgery. Furthermore the trauma and stress of the surgery itself will cause a stress response leading to catabolism and hyperglycemia and potentially

---

Features of Diabetes

Type 1

Typically presents in children & young adults
Caused by auto-immune reaction to ß cells of islets of Langerhans cells in pancreas
Insulin not formed
Insulin needed to facilitate glucose entry to cells for energy metabolism
Untreated cells metabolize fat leading to release of ketones causing keto-acidosis and death

Type 2

Usually presents age over 40 but not necessarily
Insulin level may be normal or raised but is less effective
Glucose level is increased but not as much as in type 1

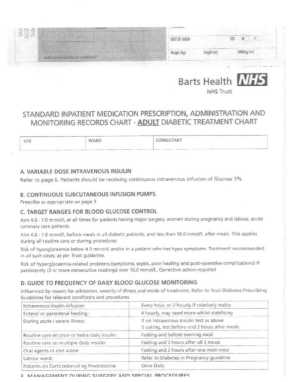

	ALLER	Side							

DATE OF BIRTH		SEX	M ☐	F ☐
Weight (kg)		Height (m)		BMI(kg/m²)

Barts Health NHS
NHS Trust

STANDARD INPATIENT MEDICATION PRESCRIPTION, ADMINISTRATION AND
MONITORING RECORDS CHART - **ADULT** DIABETIC TREATMENT CHART

SITE	WARD	CONSULTANT

A. VARIABLE DOSE INTRAVENOUS INSULIN
Refer to page 6. Patients should be receiving continuous intravenous infusion of Glucose 5%

B. CONTINUOUS SUBCUTANEOUS INFUSION PUMPS.
Prescribe as appropriate on page 3

C. TARGET RANGES FOR BLOOD GLUCOSE CONTROL
Aim 4.0 - 7.0 mmol/L at all times for patients having major surgery, women during pregnancy and labour, acute coronary care patients

Aim 4.0 - 7.0 mmol/L before meals in all diabetic patients, and less than 10.0 mmol/L after meals. This applies during all routine care or during procedures

Risk of hypoglycaemia below 4.0 mmol/L and/or in a patient who has hypo symptoms. Treatment recommended in all such cases, as per Trust guideline.

Risk of hyperglycaemia-related problems (symptoms, sepsis, poor healing and post-operative complications) if persistently (3 or more consecutive readings) over 10.0 mmol/L. Corrective action required

D. GUIDE TO FREQUENCY OF DAILY BLOOD GLUCOSE MONITORING
Influenced by reason for admission, severity of illness and mode of treatment. Refer to Trust Diabetes Prescribing Guidelines for relevant conditions and procedures

Intravenous insulin infusion:	Every hour, or 2-hourly if relatively stable
Enteral or parenteral feeding:	4 hourly, may need more whilst stabilising
During acute / severe illness:	If on intravenous insulin test as above. If eating, test before and 2 hours after meals
Routine care on once or twice daily insulin:	Fasting and before evening meal
Routine care on multiple daily insulin:	Fasting and 2 hours after all 3 meals
Oral agents or diet alone:	Fasting and 2 hours after one main meal
Labour ward:	Refer to Diabetes in Pregnancy guideline
Patients on Corticosteroid eg Prednisolone	Once Daily

E. MANAGEMENT DURING SURGERY AND SPECIAL PROCEDURES

Glucose mmol/L	Step up Stop down	customised regimen as per Diabetes Team recommendation			
< 4.0		0.5	0.5	0.5	0.5
4.0 - 6.9		1	2	3	4
7.0 - 8.9		2	4	6	8
9.0 – 10.9		3	6	9	12
11.0 – 13.9		4	8	12	16
≥ 14.0		6	12	18	24

Doctors: Prescribe from Table of Insulin Infusion Rate above

Date	Time	Scale	Signature & Contact No.

Doctor to prescribe first scale:
Start with sliding scale A, unless the patient is usually on a total daily dose of more than 100 units of insulin per day, in which case start with scale B

Do not stop patient's subcutaneous long acting insulin analogue except on the advice of the diabetes team.

Scale Adjustment by IV accredited Nurse:
If blood glucose >9.0mmol/L for more than 2 consecutive readings, STEP UP to the next scale. If scale D appears to be inadequate please contact doctor to write up custom scale.

If blood glucose <3.5mmol/L, Stop insulin for 20 minutes STEP DOWN to the next scale. Hypoglycaemia lasting for 20 minutes or more requires specialist advice.

Seek advice from Diabetes Team if unable to maintain control of BG in range 4.0 – 10.0 mmol/L bleep Diabetes Registrar via switchboard

Coming Off the Sliding Scale:
Once patient is eating and drinking normally, sliding scale may be stopped after restarting on usual diabetes treatment. Doctor to initial instructions and prescribe tablets or subcutaneous insulin on appropriate part of Diabetes chart

Monitoring after coming off sliding scale:

The inside of the chart contains simple information on dosage. In practice this will probably be written up by the anaesthetist. If you are asked to prescribe you should always ask one of your medically qualified colleagues to check it.

The Diabetic Treatment Chart is used to record the results of glucose estimations and prescribe subcutaneous insulin for diabetics in hospital. This is an adult chart; children will be on a paediatric ward and their diabetes will be managed by paediatricians.

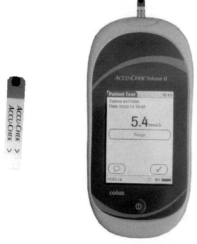

Blood glucose can be quickly tested with a blood sample taken from the end of a finger with a lancet and soaked onto a test strip (left). The strip is placed into the hand held machine (right) which gives a digital display of the result, in this case normal.

ketoacidosis. Sepsis and inflammation reduce the effectiveness of insulin produced, making control more difficult. A type 1 insulin dependent diabetic will typically need increased amounts of insulin in the peri-operative period or if systemically unwell and a type 2 non-insulin dependent diabetic may need insulin to keep their glucose levels with the ideal range (6-10 mmols./litre).

Diabetes may affect the surgery, particularly in those not well controlled. Catabolism will cause delayed wound healing. There will be an increased risk of cardio-vascular complications (myocardial infarction, heart failure and stroke), and where these complications occur mortality will be greater. Due to neuropathy myocardial infarction is more likely to be painless. Hyperglycemia will affect chemotaxis and phagocytosis and the function of polymorphonuclear leukocytes as well as acting as a culture medium; thus post-operative sepsis is more likely. Although it is less likely in OMFS, diabetic patients who are immobile in bed are more likely to develop pressure sores due to small vessel disease.

Diabetic patients presenting for cold (non-urgent) OMFS should have the standard pre-operative assessment. This will include details of any diabetic complications, how well controlled they are and blood tests for glucose, electrolytes and HbA1$_C$ (glycosylated haemoglobin). HbA1$_C$ is haemoglobin which has glucose attached to it as a result of a high blood glucose. The proportion of haemoglobin which is glycosylated gives an indication of the blood glucose over the preceding three months (the life of a red blood cell). A level of above 69 mmols./mol. or 8.5% of total haemoglobin is considered indicative of inadequate glucose control.

Patients who are well controlled, have no diabetic complications, who are having a short or minor procedure, can confidently monitor and manage their own glucose and who will miss only one meal, may be admitted as a day case or have treatment under sedation. There will be a local protocol which will involve their being treated early and reducing their daily insulin (if they are to have general anaesthesia). They will need an insulin infusion with Na and KCl during surgery. In nearly every other case they will need VRIII (variable rate intra-venous insulin infusion); this was formerly called a 'sliding scale'. There will be a separate infusion of KCl in saline and insulin with the dose varied according to hourly blood glucose levels. There will be a special chart to prescribe this and a protocol for the dose of rapidly acting insulin; the diabetic team should be informed and the diabetic team specialist nurse will visit the patient daily and decide how and when they are fit to be weaned back onto their normal regime.

Hypoglycemia

Caused by too much insulin, inadequate food intake, exercise, stress, alcohol
Can occur quickly
Most diabetics can recognise symptoms: sweating, shakiness, tachycardia, anxiety
Brain most susceptible as unable to metabolize fat leading to unconsciousness
Quickly responds to oral glucose or, if unconscious, glucagon injection
Well controlled diabetics are less able to recognize symptoms

Hyperglycemia

Associated with low intracellular glucose
Cells metabolize fat for energy producing ketones
Ketones are toxic and cause acidosis
Diabetic ketoacidosis is dangerous and causes death

Complications of Diabetes

Large vessel arteriosclerosis: myocardial infarction, stroke, peripheral vascular disease
Small vessel disease: nephropathy, retinopathy, cataracts.
Neuropathy: peripheral, autonomic

Patients who present for cold (non-urgent) surgery who are poorly controlled or have high glucose or high HbA1$_C$ should be referred to their GP for advice and management. Patients who need urgent surgery, present as emergency admissions, have complications, are poorly controlled in spite of GP care or who are regularly under the care of a diabetic specialist physician, should be monitored by the diabetic team as routine.

Key Points

• Contact diabetic team for undiagnosed diabetes or those with poor control or complications

• For cold (non-urgent) OMFS surgery – standard preoperative assessment and check HbA1c for recent glucose control

• For well controlled diabetes – consult local protocol – inform diabetic team - variable rate intra-venous insulin infusion (VRIII) or 'sliding scale', KCl in saline and hourly blood glucose check – special chart

• For poorly controlled diabetes – refer to their GP for management or diabetic physician

49. <u>Medication Related Osteonecrosis of the Jaws</u>

In 2002 we started seeing patients in our clinics who had exposed bone in the mouth with chronic discharges, pain and halitosis. This initially baffled most OMF surgeons. In April 2006 the government Chief Dental Officer advised dentists in one of his regular circular letters that the Medicines and Healthcare Products Regulatory Agency had received, through their 'yellow card' reporting system, 62 reports of these symptoms in patients who had been prescribed bisphosphonates. The association had been realised in the United States a year or so beforehand.

Bisphosphonate medication is prescribed in low doses in oral form for patients with osteopenia and osteoporosis, mostly post-menopausal women to prevent pathological fractures. It is used in higher dose through intermittent intra-venous infusions for the management of Paget's disease of bone, hypercalcaemia of malignancy, multiple myeloma and for skeletal metastases, most in women with breast cancer but also men with prostate cancer. Osteopenia and osteoporosis are common in post-menopausal women and particularly predispose to fractured neck of femur, an event which can be fatal in the frail. Many elderly ladies will be prescribed bisphosphonates when they have steroids for whatever reason as steroids decrease bone density.

The drugs work mainly by inhibiting osteoclastic bone resorption. They accumulate in bone particularly where there is a high bone turn over, as in the alveolus of the jaws. They may also inhibit tumour cells invading bone and cause tumour cell death. It is possible that bisphosphonate may be released from bone by the trauma of dental extractions and thus inhibit soft tissue healing; they may also decrease intra-bony blood circulation. There is a very high turnover of bone during remodelling after dental extraction so that symptoms are most likely to develop in this circumstance.

Bisphosphonate related osteonecrosis of the jaws has been defined as avascular necrotic bone, which may or may not be exposed, that has been present for over eight weeks in patients with no history of irradiation. However, recently a newer drug, denosumab, not a bisphosphonate, has been introduced. This interferes with osteoclast function and has been used for post-menopausal osteoporosis

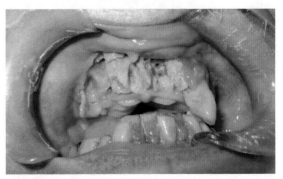

This lady presented with exposed bone in her maxilla a few weeks after she had 3 incisors removed. She has taken oral bisphosphonates along with prednisolone for polymyalgia. When she had the teeth removed it had been some time since she had taken the medication and had forgotten about it. Over the following 9 months her whole maxilla sloughed out.

and in some cases replacing bisphosphonate for cancer patients. Bevacizumab and sunitinib may be used in combination with bisphosphonates; they also contribute to necrosis. This has led to the term Medication Related Osteonecrosis of the Jaws (MRONJ) to be used.

The best estimate of the incidence of the problem comes from a study carried out by the Faculty of General Dental Practice of the Royal College of Surgeons of England and published on their web site. They report it as having an incidence of perhaps 10 patients in a million per year. It is higher in females and in the elderly. Although those taking lower dose bisphosphonates orally (most commonly alendronic acid) are less at risk than those having higher dose intermittent infusions (most commonly zoledronic acid) there are more patients with problems related to oral ingestion (56%) than IV (34%) due to the much larger number prescribed the former.

Although the incidence is rare you will see a significant number of these patients in OMFS departments as the medication is prescribed for chronic problems and patients return quite often with infective exacerbations. This applies to even the patients with metastatic breast cancer. Modern therapy and bisphosphonate means that ladies with metastatic breast cancer can lead normal lives for years. Whatever the complications (which only a

'A Curious Form of Disease'

'The disease begins with aching in a tooth that has been previously been more or less imperfect, or in people whose gums are not firmly adherent to the bone.'

'An unsound constitution... favours the development of the disease.'

'The next symptom is decaying of the jawbone. Pieces of it, probably as large as peas, work themselves out.'

'Liability to the disorder was not extremely great.'

Charles Dickens wrote these words in his journal 'Household Words' in 1852. He was describing 'phossy jaw' which affected workers exposed to phosphorus in the match industry. It was exactly the same disease as phosphorus necrosis caused by bisphosphonates 150 years later.

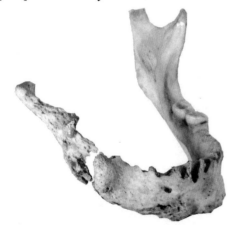

19th century mandible from match worker with phosphorus jaw necrosis. Courtesy of Royal College of Surgeons of England

small proportion get) they are wonderful drugs; hitherto metastatic breast cancer would have been crippling.

Bone necrosis itself can be asymptomatic but when it becomes infected swelling, pain and discharge develop. In most cases this is precipitated by dental extraction although it can occur from denture trauma, particularly on the thin mucosa lingually in the lower molar area or over tori. The longer a patient has been on the medication the greater the risk; most of those on oral bisphosphonate have taken it for three years before getting symptoms.

So what do we do for patients who need dental extractions and are on bisphosphonates and how are those with established necrosis managed? As the disease has only been known for just over a decade there is no clear universally accepted guideline so you may find management is different in different departments. However there are some patterns of accepted practice emerging.

It is generally accepted that patients should be made dentally fit before starting the drugs. Your hospital may have a fast track system for patients to be assessed before they start medication (particularly IV) and any non-restorable teeth removed and the socket allowed to heal for three weeks before the first dose. Our experience has shown that OMFS referral and subsequent treatment prior to bisphosphonate therapy keeps the risk of bone necrosis low.

Good oral hygiene support and restorative care should be provided by someone, and smoking should be advised against. Patients on oral bisphosphonates are at lower risk especially if taking the drug for a short time. They may have extractions carried out as atraumatically as possible and sharp socket edges burred back without raising a muco-periosteal flap. Patients taking oral drugs for over three years and particularly those taking steroids should be warned of higher risk. It has been considered that cessation of the bisphosphonates may be helpful but the drugs bind to bone so well that it is considered that stopping for anything less than a year before extractions would probably not be helpful. Denosumab does not bind into the skeleton like bisphosphonates so ceasing the drug will allow the effect on osteoclasts to recover so that its effects are reversible in time. Stopping steroids is considered to produce an immediate reduction in risk and if this is not possible then reducing the dose to below 7.5 mgs. per day may help. Preoperative and post-operative oral chlorhexidine mouth rinses may help but antibiotics probably not, unless there is active sepsis before.

Patients on IV bisphosphonates should avoid extractions wherever feasible. For unrestorable teeth removing the crown and root filling the root has been advocated. Otherwise advice is as above.

Patients who have osteonecrosis may be asymptomatic with exposed bone in the mouth. Some have advocated covering exposed bone with local flaps but generally they should be managed as conservatively as possible, keeping the area clean with

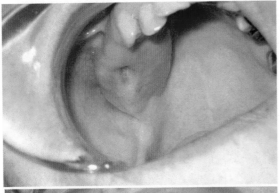

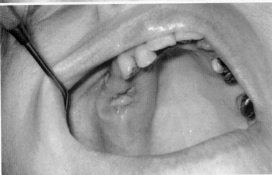

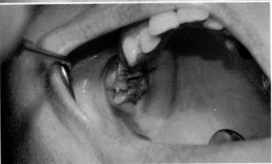

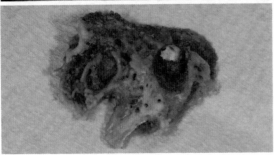

Risk factors for bone necrosis

↑ risk IV bisphosphonates than oral

↑ mandible than the maxilla

↑ periodontal disease

↑ steroids

↑ immunosuppressants or chemotherapy

↑ poorly controlled diabetes

↑ smoking

↑ combination with Bevacizumab or Sunitinib

chlorhexidine without brushing the delicate soft tissues and exposing more bone. When the exposed bone becomes infected they will get swelling, pain, discharge and halitosis. Acute exacerbations may be managed with penicillin based antibiotics, or metronidazole. Bone concentrating antibiotics such as tetracycline or clindamycin may be useful as may pentoxifylline a local vasodilator which is commonly used to improve blood supply in intermittent claudication. Calcichew provides calcium as does alfacalcidol a type of vitamin D. However chronic sepsis for months or years is the norm; if the sepsis is draining it may be painless, just sore. Some may advocate removing large bony sequestra and infected necrotic bone and covering with local flaps but surgery may increase the risk of pathological fracture.

In cases where the mandible is discharging pus extra-orally or where there is a pathological fracture a segmental resection of the mandible may be considered but reconstruction will be difficult because all the bone will be abnormal; there will be no normal bone to attach a graft to. In general, surgery has the possibility of making an awkward or difficult clinical situation an awful lot worse so a mature surgeon will be wary of operating only on patients already in extremis.

A typical case. This lady was able to have a normal lifestyle for many years in spite of metastatic breast cancer thanks to her monthly bisphosphonate infusions. She presented with discharge after removal of her upper first molar. The images show the alveolar bone extruding over a period of 2 years. After the socket was exfoliated pus continued to discharge.

50. <u>Anticoagulation and Surgery</u>

Many patients are receiving anticoagulant therapy because they are at risk of thromboembolism due to atrial fibrillation, previous thrombosis or because they have mechanical heart valves. Most of them will be receiving the coumarin drug warfarin which works by blocking the formation of prothrombin and clotting factors 2, 7, 9 and 10. It prevents the metabolism of vitamin K to its active form for synthesis of these factors. Warfarin binds strongly to plasma proteins so it has a long half-life of about 36 hours which means the full anti-coagulant effects take some time to be reached and continue for several days after the medication is stopped.

The degree of anticoagulation is measured with the prothrombin test and is expressed as the INR (International Normalized Ratio) which is the ratio of the prothrombin time divided by a laboratory control. An INR of 1 would be normal, i.e. no anti-coagulation, and 2 would mean the blood would take twice as long to clot. Patients have their warfarin doses adjusted to achieve the INR appropriate to the problem they have which might lead to thromboembolism. This will be between 2 and 3 for patients at risk due to atrial fibrillation, a previous deep vein thrombosis or pulmonary embolism or transient ischemic events or strokes. A higher ratio of between 3 and 4 is appropriate for those who are at risk because of heart valve disorders including mechanical heart valves or a recent myocardial infarct.

It has been shown that patients who are anti-coagulated within these therapeutic ranges of INR 2-4 are likely to have some additional risk of bleeding over those who are not anti-coagulated if they have minor oral surgery including dental extractions. However when they do bleed this is nearly always susceptible to being stopped by simple local measures such as packing, suturing and tranexamic acid used locally. Stopping the anticoagulation places them at increased risk of rebound thrombosis so it is generally recommended that no adjustment is appropriate if the patient's INR is within the therapeutic range (INR <4).

Patients who take warfarin will have an anti-coagulant card with all their blood results on it. If they have a stable result they should not need to come to hospital for dental extractions. However some patients will have confounding factors which put them at additional risk such as an unstable and variable INR,

additional disease processes which might affect their coagulation such as liver disease, renal failure, other coagulopathy or history of alcohol abuse. Some patients may be taking additional medication which may potentiate warfarin such as anti-hypertensives, antifungals, carbamazepine, steroids, phenytoin, aspirin, and antibiotics such as erythromycin and metronidazole. In these situations treatment in hospital will give the patient greater confidence that should excess bleeding occur measures will be quickly available to help.

In all cases oral wounds should be packed with oxidized cellulose gauze and sutured with absorbable sutures. If bleeding persists locally applied tranexamic acid will be helpful. In the very unusual situation where an anti-coagulated patient continues to bleed after local measures have been applied help from a haematologist should be requested. Warfarin can be reversed with intravenous vitamin K or with fresh frozen plasma. Reversal with vitamin K is slower and has the disadvantage that there may be later resistance to warfarin. Reversal with fresh frozen plasma is immediate and does not have this problem.

Occasionally a patient on warfarin may present as an emergency with facial injuries. In this case the haematologist should be involved as the patient will probably need the anticoagulation reversing if there is persistent bleeding. If the patient does not appear to be actively bleeding or it has stopped it would be prudent to inform the haematologist of the patient's existence in case a problem develops.

Sometimes an anti-coagulated patient will need more extensive surgery. This is most likely to be an elderly patient who needs cancer ablation which may involve a neck dissection where post-operative haemorrhage is potentially dangerous. Here the warfarin should be reduced over 4 or 5 days before, until the INR is about 1.5. In this case the increased risk of thromboembolism will have to be accepted. In patients where the risk is highest, such as those with a recent thromboembolic event, the anti-coagulation can be replaced by 'bridging therapy' with sub-cutaneous injections of low molecular weight heparin (enoxaparin). Low molecular weight heparin has a half-life of only a few hours and its effect can be reversed with protamine. In a very few cases it will be necessary for the patient to receive intra-venous heparin with the dose being adjusted monitored by APPT testing.

It has been suggested that patients taking anti-coagulants should not receive inferior dental nerve blocks because of the risk of serious bleeding into the medial pterygoid muscle. There has been no scientific proof that this is the case and we have never seen a case where this has been a problem.

Recently newer anticoagulant drugs sometimes termed 'target specific' or 'novel' anticoagulants have been developed which have certain advantages over warfarin for long term anti-coagulation. Dabigatran etixilate is a direct thrombin inhibitor and rivaroxaban, apixaban and edoxaban are factor 10a inhibitors. These drugs have much shorter half-lives than warfarin so they have a more rapid onset of action after oral ingestion and a much quicker offset, provided the patient does not have renal failure. They have a lower risk of unwanted bleeding, few drug interactions, much reduced variability of effect between individuals, and do not require anti-coagulant monitoring; indeed there is no reliable test to do so. On the negative side there is no effective way of reversing their effect other than by stopping the medication. However idarucizumab, a newer drug which is a humanised antibody fragment, has been recently developed which binds to dabigatran and neutralises its anticoagulant effect and can therefore be used in an emergency situation.

It was only in 2012 that dabigatran received approval from the National Institute of Clinical Excellence for thrombo-prophylaxis for stroke and patients with atrial fibrillation (not accompanied by valve disease). It is therefore too soon for a definitive experience to have been established on how patients taking these drugs should be managed during surgery. However it would appear that patients requiring dental extraction and minor oral surgery do not suffer any major problems if these drugs are continued as normal. It is recommended that ideally the surgery should be carried out 12 hours after the last dose, wounds should be sutured and that the patient should rinse with 5% tranexamic acid for a few days after the surgery.

At present drugs for the reversal of these anticoagulants are only in development, apart from dabigatran, so it would be prudent that patients who need more major surgery should have them temporarily discontinued and re-started afterwards. Obviously this management should be supervised in hospital by a specialist haematologist.

Although not anticoagulants we would like to mention antiplatelet medication with Aspirin, clopidogrel and dipyridamole. These drugs are used to prevent platelet adhesion and prevent unwanted vascular events such as acute coronary thrombosis, stroke and transient ischemic attacks. For minor oral surgery such as surgical dental extraction the risk of bleeding which cannot be controlled by local measures is very low so surgery should proceed without stopping the medication.

However for more major surgery each case should be considered on its own merit; there is little in the way of clinical trials to help firm guidelines to be formulated. If medication is to be ceased it will need to be done several days in advance as the drugs have half-lives of several days. The decision should be made by the senior surgeon in discussion with the haematologist as in some cases this may be potentially dangerous. Some patients who have had 'drug eluting stents' fitted to prevent coronary artery occlusion are at serious risk of thrombosis if their combined Aspirin and clopidogrel therapy is stopped. In such cases the cardiologist should be involved in the decision with the Consultant surgeon. You should never make the decision to stop medication yourself.

Key Points

- For MOS for patients on Warfarin check INR is stable

- Proceed if below 4, pack wound with oxidised cellulose gauze and suture

- Patients on 'novel anticoagulants' proceed as normal and pack and suture as above

- Patients on clopidogrel, aspirin or dipyridamole proceed as normal for MOS

- For more major surgery involve haematologist.

- Never stop medication on your own volition

51. <u>Understanding Orthognathic Surgery</u>

Correction of facial deformity can be complicated and involve many different surgical procedures; craniofacial surgery which involves high level facial osteotomies on syndromic youngsters is normally carried out in a few craniofacial units which have sufficient numbers of these unusual cases to maintain the specialist expertise. However, orthognathic surgery (correction of jaw disproportion) is common, fairly simple and carried out in most OMFS departments with one operation, the bimaxillary osteotomy, colloquially known as the 'bimax'. This consists of a maxillary osteotomy at Le Fort 1 level and a sagittal split osteotomy of the mandible, colloquially know as a 'sag'.

Although there are a handful of cases carried out to improve the airway in patients with obstructive sleep apnoea most cases will be young adults who have a severe bony discrepancy in their dental base relationships and a malocclusion which cannot be corrected by orthodontics alone. Treatment will normally involve 12 – 24 months of pre-surgical orthodontics followed by surgery and approximately 6 months of orthodontic retention before everything is complete.

The whole process will involve many orthodontic visits in addition to a major surgical operation, so a lot of commitment is needed both from the patient and their family. The patients are generally highly motivated as they are anticipating an improvement in facial appearance in addition to a functional occlusion with stable oral health. Many youngsters with facial or jaw disproportion will be affected psychologically by their appearance and may have experienced teasing or bullying at school. Some OMFS departments may have a clinical psychologist attached to their teams but we are unsure of what the benefit is as it is the orthodontics and surgery that improves their well-being and confidence.

The surgery, which results in discomfort (rather than frank pain), difficulty eating, some time with jaws held together, and a change in appearance, is a major life event for most. It is frequently carried out at the age of 17 when growth has finished; in order that it should interfere with education as little as possible this is often at the end of school year before the start of higher education. The end of June through to the beginning of August is a busy time for the orthognathic surgeon.

Class 3 before orthodontics

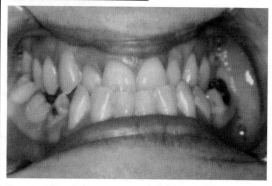

Pre-treatment. There is a reverse overjet with the lower incisors in front of the uppers and the lower buccal segments are wider than the upper.

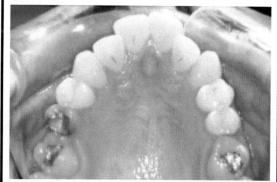

Pre-treatment. The upper arch is irregular.

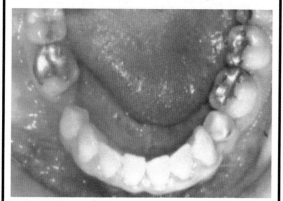

Pre-treatment. The lower incisors are obviously retroclined as well as there being irregularities.

Most cases will follow one of two patterns: the class 3 case, which is the most common, and the class 2 division 1. In the class 3 case the mandible will be prognathic compared to the maxilla. The maxillary buccal segments will be too narrow, and the upper incisors will be proclined towards the mandibular incisors which will be retroclined by the soft tissues towards the maxillary. The incisor relationship will be class 3 or just edge to edge. Facially the patient will have an obvious prominent mandible, the maxilla will appear flat in profile and long so that there will be more than the ideal 2 mm incisor show when the mouth is at rest and the patient may show a variable amount of gingiva when smiling rather than the lip moving only to the gingival margin.

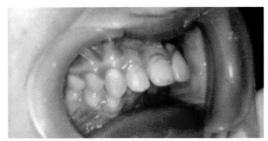

Class 2 div. 1

In the class 2 division 1 case the patient will have an obvious mandibular deficiency in profile with upper incisors proclined by the lower lip which fits inside them and over-erupted lower incisors producing a significantly increased curve of Spee to the occlusion; the lower incisors may be traumatising the palatal gingiva.

Children with bony jaw discrepancies should be seen by the orthodontist early as they can often influence growth patterns using treatment with extra-oral headgear. In cases where the patient will need surgery to correct their disproportion they should be seen by the orthodontist and surgeon together with their parents before surgery is contemplated. A dental examination, orthopantomograph and lateral cephalometric X-rays are carried out and study models taken. After these examinations the recommendations concerning possible surgery can be made and considered by the patient. These steps are normally carried out over several visits. When recommendations are made it is essential that the patient is informed of all the potential complications and side effects of the treatment, both orthodontic and surgical, and consent for the treatment obtained and recorded in writing. It is helpful if all this information is put in writing in the form of a letter to the patient, with copies to the primary care practitioners, and a copy kept with the written confirmation of consent. It is also helpful for the patient to meet someone who has already undergone surgery.

Apart from an orthopantomograph X-ray a lateral cephalometric X-ray is made. This involves an image taken with the X-ray source some distance away from the patient and sensor so that the rays are near parallel. This image can then be traced to measure angles of the face and dentition and facial height, and to predict the final result for the patient. However we have some reservations about prediction as it is not always accurate. We are nervous about disappointing a patient if the appearance is not as they feel they had been promised. It is imperative that before orthodontics is started that the patient is motivated to achieve high standards of oral hygiene and sensible diet as the pre-surgical orthodontics will take between one and two years with fixed appliances.

In the common class 3 case the aim of orthodontics is to correct any irregularity in the occlusion, expand the maxillary buccal segments and de-compensate the incisor tilting so that the upper incisors are near the normal 109° to the maxillary plane and the lower incisors are 90° to the mandibular plane. This will make the facial appearance worse initially; the patient should have been warned about it.

In class 2 cases where the mandible is to be moved forward the orthodontics will also need to help flatten the curve of Spee and tilt the incisors in the opposite direction to that of a class 3 case. If the lower incisors have erupted significantly then the lower labial segment may be set down at surgery in which case orthodontics can create a small space between the canines and premolars to make room for a bone cut. Surgery for class 2 cases often involves a genioplasty to put the chin forward to help mask the skeletal discrepancy if this is severe.

Before the orthodontics has been completed the patient should be seen again by a surgeon and a date set for surgery. The procedure should be explained to them again and they should be warned about side effects and complications and the final movements are planned. The orthodontist will order a new lateral cephalometric X-ray image which will be traced digitally to help with the planning, and new study models will be made to be mounted on an articulator.

One of the potential complications of this type of surgery is relapse. That is to say that the soft tissues,

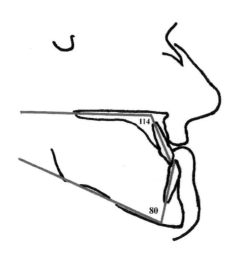

Before: The soft tissues have 'compensated' the incisor relationship for the discrepancy in the dental base relationship. The tongue has tilted the upper incisors forward to an angulation of 114° to the maxillary plane (norm: 109°) and the lip has tilted the lower incisor back to an angulation of 80° to the mandibular plane (norm: 90°).

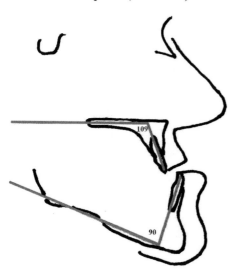

After: The incisors have been 'decompensated' to the normal angulation ready for surgery. The patient should be warned of the temporary adverse effect on facial profile.

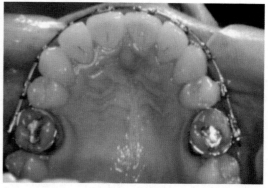

The upper arch has been expanded and irregularities removed. The incisors have been retroclined towards the norm of 108° to the maxillary plane.

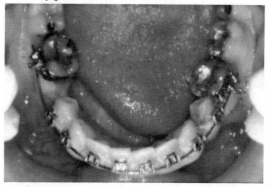

The lower incisors have been inclined forward to bring the lower incisor to mandibular place angle towards the norm of 90°.

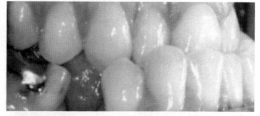

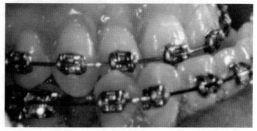

After pre-surgical orthodontics the incisor relation will look worse (above before, below after).

muscles, ligaments have a habit of pulling the bony skeleton back to where it used to be. Patients should be warned that in many cases there will be a very small amount of relapse in the years after surgery but in a few cases the relapse may be severe. Having a well-fitting positive occlusion will help stability as will keeping the movements to a minimum by equalising the correction of the discrepancy between both maxilla and mandible. Thus in most cases patients will have surgery to both jaws: the 'bimax'.

Generally the orthodontist will prescribe the movements to be made using the cephalometric tracings to analyse the facial skeleton. However any competent OMFS surgeon will be able to prescribe the movements to be made from clinical examination as follows:-

First look at the patient in profile and see if there is any flat appearance of the face (para-nasal flattening) and what the angle is between the upper lip and alar of the nose (90° norm). Then decide if the maxilla needs to be advanced to get the optimal facial appearance: not at all, a little (3mm), a medium amount (6 mm) or a lot (9 mm). Next observe the face from in front: does it look long? Observe the amount of incisor show with the lips at rest (2 mm norm) and when the patient is smiling (lips to top of clinical crown). This assumes a normal lip length of 22 mm for males and 20 mm for females. Then decide if the maxilla needs to be impacted surgically, not at all, a little (2mms), a medium amount (4 mm) or a lot (6 mm). We like to compare our conclusion made by clinical examination with that of the orthodontists made radiographically; the result is nearly always within a mm or so. It is a nonsense to measure differential distances in single millimetres; the surgical technique is simply not that accurate.

The models are then mounted on an articular by the technician who then carries out model surgery to the maxilla and makes the movements prescribed and constructs a wafer to fit between the teeth after the maxilla has been moved and before the mandible. This ''intermediate wafer' is used by the surgeon to position the maxilla after making the cuts while it is plated firmly into position. The mandible is then moved into a class 1 relationship to the maxilla and a wafer made to hold the mandible firmly in position with the jaws wired together while the surgeon plates the mandible.

Surgery takes from just over an hour for a single jaw operation and up to four and a half hours for a bimaxillary procedure. Patients should be warned that

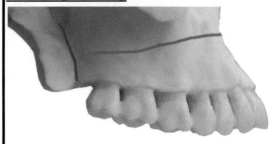

Bimaxillary osteotomy

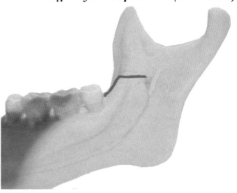

The pterygoid plates are disconnected from the maxilla with a curved chisel placed behind the maxilla (blue line), the buccal maxilla is cut with a bur or saw through the lateral wall of the nose (anteriorly) and lateral wall of antrum (posteriorly-red line) and the nasal septum is divided with a chisel using only hand pressure (not shown).

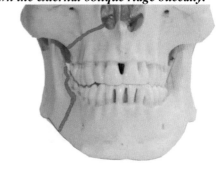

The mandible cortex is cut medially (red line) through to bleeding cancellous bone within just just above the lingua, so avoiding the ID bundle (yellow), and only half way back and is continued down the external oblique ridge buccally.

The cortical cut is extended down and through the cortical bone at the lower border. The cuts top and bottom are then gently opened with a large chisel and the maxilla downfractured and the mandible split sagittally.

they may need up to three nights in hospital but in practice only one is normally required.

Although the jaws are plated with titanium plates they are normally approximated together with inter-maxillary elastic bands. This is done because the patient will have to re-learn the proprioception necessary to close the mandible into a correct occlusive position. The elastics may be placed the day after the operation or a few days later at the first follow up appointment. Patients are normally given steroids during the peri-operative period. This helps reduce the amount of oedematous swelling, reduce nausea and the amount of analgesia needed. It also delays swelling so they must be warned that they will swell further in the couple of days following surgery before it starts to go down. Once surgery is over the patient will probably need a few further months with an orthodontic appliance to help retain the teeth in the new positions.

We hope that you will be able to participate in the treatment of orthognathic patients. You should make sure you have the opportunity to interview and examine any patient whose operation you assist with and be able to see them in the clinic during the post-operative period in order to appreciate what this interesting and rewarding surgery has to offer. With increasing specialisation there are now many surgeons who do little other than orthognathic surgery; this has the advantage that they are able to offer less frequently performed operations for more unusual deformities. The vast majority of cases, however continue to be managed with simple 'bimax'.

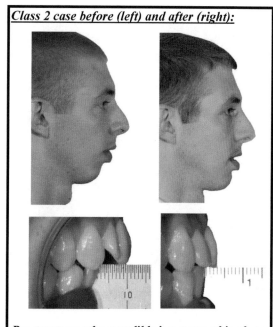

Class 3 case before (left) and after (right):

Pre-treatment the mandible is prognathic, the maxilla looks slightly flat beside the nose, there is a reverse overjet of 3 mms.

Class 2 case before (left) and after (right):

Pre-treatment the mandible is retrognathic, there is an overjet of 9 mms.

Side effects of surgery

Swelling
Bruising
Jaws fixed together
Discomfort eating
Weight Loss
Temporary numbness or tingling of lip or chin

Complications of Surgery

Permanent numbness of lip or chin (approx 30%)
Relapse
Infection of bone plates necessitating surgery for removal

52. __Introduction to Facial Skin Cancer__

Surgery for facial skin cancer has been increasingly carried out in OMFS departments in recent years. It was traditionally the work of plastic surgeons, who still do most of this work; however there is plenty for everyone. The majority of the patients are elderly and pleasant, the surgery is not taxing and most cases are very suitable for outpatient operations, carried out using local anaesthetic in a dental chair.

We include this topic to help the core dental trainee understand the work of the speciality. Also as dental surgeons spend their practising careers looking at faces and as skin cancer is more common than all the other major cancers together, it is a good thing for them to understand and be able to recognise the disease.

Cancer of the skin (squamous and basal carcinoma and malignant melanoma), is responsible for about 20% of all new cancer cases reported in the UK; however only a very small proportion of the deaths. Malignant melanoma compromises about 10% of skin cancer cases but is responsible for most of the skin cancer deaths.

There has been an increasing incidence of skin cancer over the last few decades, the main culprit being ultra-violet radiation mostly from sunlight, but also artificial. The other risk factors are increasing age, family history, multiple moles, fair skin which tends to burn easily on exposure to the sun, and patients taking immunosuppressants.

As with all cancers treatment should be undertaken as part of a multidisciplinary team which includes surgeons, an oncologist, pathologist, a clinical nurse specialist and, most importantly, a dermatologist. The initial referral from the primary care physician should ideally be to the dermatologist who will be able, in most cases, to make a confident diagnosis clinically without histology; this is not the case with most other

__Suspect malignant melanoma if:__
A:- Asymmetrical
B:- Border irregular
C:- Colour not uniform
D:- Diameter more than 6 mms
E:- Evolving

__Basal Cell Carcinoma__

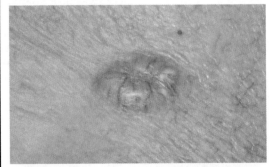

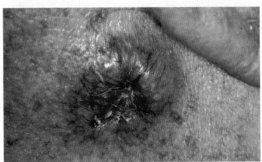

Above are examples of the most common, nodular type. It is a pearly translucent papule or nodule with a central depression or crater, telangiectasia and a rolled waxy margin.

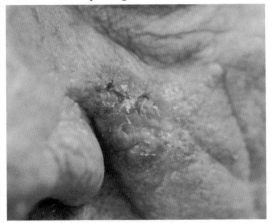

The least common morphoeic BCC is atrophic, white, slightly eroded or crusted plaque often looking like a scar. It is the most aggressive and difficult to treat as it is very difficult to define the margins. This lesion is very suitable for treatment with Mohs micrographic surgery or radiotherapy.

174

cancers. Often they will use a dermatoscope which uses polarised light to produce a very clear image which is magnified and can be recorded.

Dermatologists often carry out curettage of very small squamous and basal cells carcinomas, a technique not normally used by surgeons. The soft cancer is scraped out with a curette and requires some considerable experience to differentiate, by feel, the cancer tissue from normal skin. Pre-malignant lesions may be managed by freezing with liquid nitrogen spray or topical chemotherapy using 5-fluorouracil, diclofenac gel or imiquimod. Dermatologists may also carry out simple surgery of cases which require an elliptical incision with direct closure and refer only larger lesions which need flap repair or grafts; however some dermatologists may do this surgery themselves.

Most facial skin cancers can be excised with a simple elliptical incision and closed directly. The direction of 'Relaxed Skin Tension Lines' should be taken into account when planning the incision; the length of ellipse should be three times its width to ensure easy closure. Quite large lesions may be removed by this technique particularly because most patients are elderly and have quite lax skin which can be undermined and therefore easily stretched. Larger wounds may be closed with transposition flaps of skin from an adjacent area or full thickness skin grafts often taken from behind or in front of the ear or from the neck. Some wounds in areas difficult to close, such as the scalp, may be allowed to heal by secondary intention (as long as there is still periosteum covering the bone). Local flaps may be 'random pattern' where the blood supply is dependent upon small randomly orientated subcutaneous blood vessels or 'axial pattern' where the tissue is based on an artery which brings it's blood supply so the length can be much longer without compromising the perfusion of the tip.

Mohs micrographic surgery is a technique normally carried out by surgical dermatologists for larger malignant or pre-malignant lesions with a high risk of recurrence due to poorly defined margins, histological type or location. Lesions in the central face around the eyes, nose or mouth generally have a poorer prognosis. In Mohs technique the lesion is removed in stages with a pathologist examining specimens from the periphery of the wound using frozen sections, over a number of hours, or paraffin wax sections over a number of days. This approach is intensive in labour and hence expense but has been shown to produce very high cure rates. Once the dermatologist and pathologist are confident that all the lesion has been

Squamous Cell Carcinoma

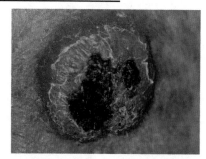

The lesion is hard with a rolled edge and ulcerated on the surface which has been bleeding.

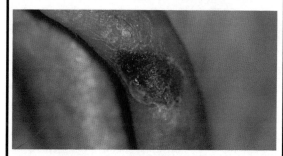

An early lesion on the outer helix of the ear in sun-damaged skin.

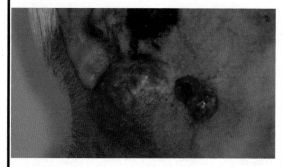

SCC of the ear has a habit of metastasing to the lymph nodes within the parotid many years later.

Relaxed Skin Tension Lines

These correspond to orientation of collagen in dermis and are parallel to underlying muscle fibres.

Where possible surgical incisions should be made in the direction of the lines to produce better healing with less scarring.

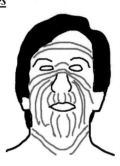

removed the resulting defect can be referred for reconstructive surgery using soft tissue flaps.

Surgical treatment has the lowest overall failure rate for facial skin cancer although radiotherapy may be useful as an adjuvant treatment for larger squamous or recurrent multiple basal cell carcinomas or as a primary treatment where a patient is unable to tolerate surgery. Radiotherapy is generally less convenient, has the risk of radionecrosis and produces an inferior cosmetic result, although this is seldom an issue for older patients. Should a radiotherapy treated lesion recur it cannot be used a second time and any subsequent surgery will be compromised by tissue damage and healing will be prolonged.

Malignant melanoma is radio resistant. Treatment should be primarily excising the lesion with a wide local margin after the case has been discussed by the skin cancer multidisciplinary team.

It is essential with all surgical procedures that all cancerous tissue is removed. In cases where the surgeon is not sure the wound can be dressed and reconstructed at a later date or further tissue removed after the pathology specimen has been examined. This particularly suits skin grafting or leaving the wound to heal by secondary intention.

Nomenclature

Papule: A circumscribed solid elevation of skin

Nodule: A palpable solid lesion in the skin or subcutaneous tissue, it extends deeper than a papule

Macule: A circumscribed flat area of discolouration without elevation or depression of surface

Plaque: A well-circumscribed, elevated, superficial, solid lesion, greater than 1 cm in diameter

Nevus: A circumscribed benign overgrowth of tissues which are normally present in the skin

In-situ: A lesion which contains malignant cells that have not metastasised or extended beyond the epidermis

Telangectasia: small dilated blood vessels visible near the surface

Malignant Melanoma

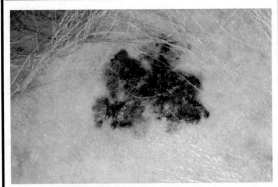

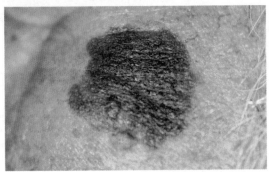

Above are examples of nodular malignant melanoma. They have irregular margins and pigmentation in varying shades of brown and black. The malignant cells grow up to form nodules and down to invade sub-dermal tissues, regional and distant lymph nodes and eventually liver, lungs and brain.

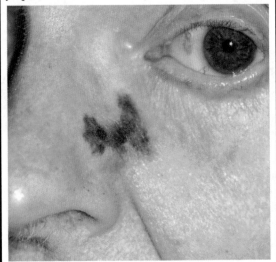

Superficial spreading melanoma grows horizontally rather than vertically down. It is macular or only slightly palpable.

Lentigo Maligna

Also known as Hutchinson's freckle, it is analogous to pre-malignant change in the oral mucosa, an 'in-situ' malignant melanoma.

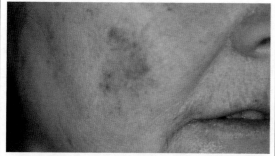

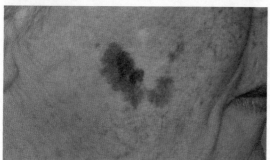

Two examples of lentigo maligna. Note the varying colour. Biopsies from different parts of the lesion will show variable change so the lesions require complete removal often needing extensive surgery (for a lesion which might not become frankly invasive anyway).

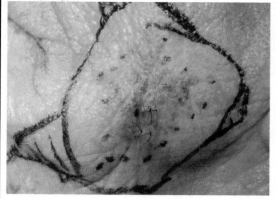

The black area within this facial lentigo maligna is nodular malignant melanoma arising. The dots mark the visible extent of the lesion and the continuous line the extent of the resection about to be undertaken.

Benign lesions

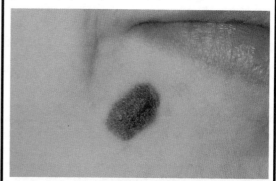

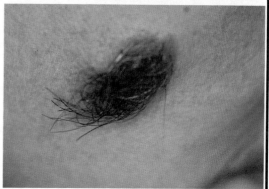

Melanocytic nevi may be congenital or acquired. They vary greatly in appearance and may be flat, elevated, smooth, rough, sessile or polyp like. Symmetric shape, regular border, uniform colour and small size suggest these lesions are benign. The lower one is intradermal (it has hair). Bleeding or a change in size, colour or shape are suspicious of malignancy.

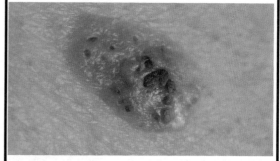

Seborrhoeic keratosis are entirely benign, they mostly occur from middle age onwards so that most elderly people have some. Pigmentation is variable, some may be very dark and if flat may appear like a melanoma. No treatment is necessary.

53. <u>Understanding Potentially Malignant Oral Disorders</u>

A vast number of patients each year will be referred to oral & maxillofacial departments because they have lesions in the mouth which are potentially malignant. These are erythroplakia (which are red patches which are often dysplastic, and often transform into malignancy), leukoplakia (which are white and approximately 30% may become malignant), mixed red and white lesions, oral sub-mucous fibrosis and lichen planus (which has the potential to become malignant but has a very low transformation rate). Overall the prevalence of these lesions may be between 0.2 to 11 %, depending on which study is the most accurate, and they have been reported as having an overall rate of transformation of between 1 and 30%.

These lesions represent a challenge because they are large in number and the majority will never become malignant. We need to decide which of these should be followed up and if there is any intervention we can make which will improve the prognosis of those that will.

In most cases a clinical diagnosis may be made after taking a full clinical and medical history combined with clinical examination. The history should always include a full medical, medication, allergy history as well as enquiry about smoking, drinking and chewing habits and presence of skin lesions. Examination should include palpation for cervical lymph nodes and examination of all of the oral mucosa with a good light and palpation of the lesion(s) with a gloved finger and a note of oral hygiene and any sharp or uneven teeth or prostheses.

Some white patches (or ulcers) on the buccal mucosa or tongue may be frictional from sharp or broken teeth. Removal of the cause will allow resolution of the problem but be aware that sharp teeth can rub cancers as well as normal mucosa and that careful follow up or immediate biopsy of the lesion is essential to be reassured of a benign diagnosis.

Lichen Planus Types of Lesion
Reticular
Plaques
Atrophic
Erosive
Desquamative gingivitis
Bullous

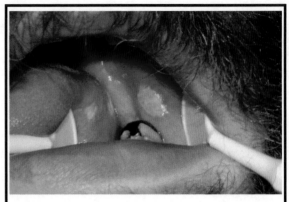

Lichenoid reactions can occur to dental restorative material composites, gold, cobalt or most commonly amalgam as here. This may be a sensitivity to amalgam but patch testing is generally unhelpful. Removing the filling and replacement with an alternative material is often rewarded with a resolution or improvement of the lesion but is not guaranteed.

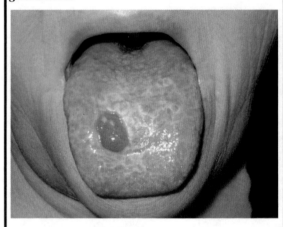

A florid lichen planus of the tongue with a granulation in an erosion.

Most white patches in the mouth will be oral lichen planus, a chronic cell mediated immune condition of unknown cause leading to hyperkeratosis; it occurs mostly in females of late middle age. Most cases will be asymptomatic and no treatment is necessary or possible and the clinical issue, particularly for the plaque like patches, is which ones to biopsy to exclude dysplasia or malignancy or to confirm the diagnosis. The typical histological appearance is of lymphocytic infiltration into the superficial connective tissue and liquefaction degeneration of the basal cells. Lichen planus does not contain evidence of dysplasia. The term 'lichenoid dysplasia' is used when a dysplastic lesion is accompanied by a dense lymphocytic response is seen in the sub-epithelial connective tissue layer like lichen planus.

Except in the case of betel quid chewers (betel leaf, tobacco, slaked lime and areca nut) there is a low incidence of malignancy in the buccal mucosa so we believe that in the very common circumstance of obvious reticular lichen planus at this site the patient may be reassured of the diagnosis without biopsy and no follow up arranged, with the patient advised to return if symptoms occur or there is a change in appearance. For plaque like and ulcerative lesions a biopsy will be necessary to make a diagnosis and if lichen planus is diagnosed follow up for a couple of years may be prudent, with further review by the primary care doctor or dentist after that. There is, however, no evidence that this will be effective in either early diagnosis of or survival from a possible squamous cancer.

Leukoplakia is a clinical diagnosis made for a white patch which cannot be wiped off, and for which another diagnosis which has not increased risk of cancer has been excluded. Thus an acute pseudomembranous candidiasis will be excluded as it can be wiped off as will white spongy nevus, frictional keratosis, habitual lip and cheek biting, chemical burn, leukoedema, lichen planus, lichenoid reaction, hairy leucoplakia, smoker's keratosis of the palate and obviously a skin graft.

It is probable that the risk of malignant change is greater in lesions which are large, cover several oral mucosal surfaces, are situated on the floor of the mouth or ventral surface of the tongue, are infected with candida hyphae, are thick and non-homogeneous (rather than thin and uniform) and particularly if they are speckled containing red areas. Proliferative verrucous leucoplakia with multiple foci and covering a wide area is considered the worst clinical appearance for malignant change. Risk factors for developing a potentially malignant leukoplakia are tobacco, alcohol and betel quid chewing. The risk of malignant transformation may be greater in older females and if the patient has extensive lesions not associated with smoking and high alcohol intake.

These lesions should always be investigated with a biopsy. The presence of dysplasia is a prognostic indicator of potential malignant change. Dysplasia is graded as mild, moderate or severe but the grading is inexact with much inter- and intra-observer variation. A mild dysplasia can be reversed if a patient with a

---

> ### *Grading of Dysplasia*
>
> *Mild*
> Limited to lower ⅓ of epithelium
> Minimal atypia
>
> *Moderate*
> Extends to middle ⅓ of epithelium
> Mild atypia extending to middle ⅓
>
> *Severe*
> Greater than ⅔ of epithelium
> Atypia in more than ⅔ of epithelium
>
> *Grading is inexact and depends principally on:*
>
> *Architecture of epithelium (irregular stratification, loss of polarity of basal cells, drop-shaped rete ridges, increased mitotic figures, abnormal superficial mitoses, keratin pearls in rete ridges. And secondarily: Cell atypia (variation in cell size and shape, nucleus size, shape and number and atypical mitotic figures.*

---

smoking or alcohol habit can be persuaded to stop, but not necessarily. For severe dysplasias surgical excision, often with a carbon dioxide laser, is frequently carried out. This is considered to reduce the incidence of, or delay, malignant change. It is not carried out for mild dysplasia and for moderate dysplasia it may not be beneficial. For very large lesions excision can be a formidable problem. The alternative is to carefully observe the lesions as malignant change is far from inevitable. One problem to consider is that a leucoplakia is probably not homogenous histologically and one part of the lesion may have mild or moderate dysplasia and another part may have a micro-invasive carcinoma or carcinoma-in-situ (cancer that does not extend beyond the epithelium). There are techniques such as staining with toluidine blue, cytology with a brush biopsy and optical techniques which are alleged to predict the dysplasia but we believe these are yet to be fully evaluated. There is evidence that staining with Lugol's iodine before laser excision of dysplasia may show up dysplasia beyond the visible margin and this will facilitate wider excision which in turn will decrease recurrence of the lesion and malignant transformation.

Where possible, removal of the entire lesion with a carbon dioxide laser will allow histological examination of all of the lesion and if dysplasia is present will stop malignant change in (possibly) half of cases but not all; so long term follow up is essential.

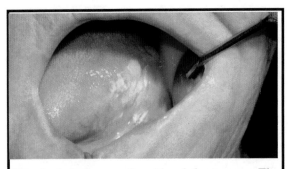

Dysplasic lesion on the side of the tongue. The tongue should always be regarded with suspicion. Removal of the lesion with CO_2 will allow all the lesion to be analyzed by the pathologist (in case it contains a small, micro-invasive cancer or carcinoma-in-situ) but will not necessarily reduce the risk of malignant change. Careful advice and follow up is desirable.

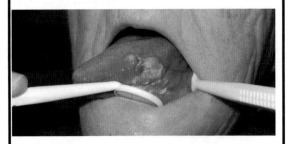

The same patient 3 years later; a cancer has arisen in the lesion. The sutures are from the biopsy.

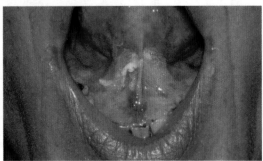

Floor of mouth keratosis has a high potential for malignant transformation.

However, many patients will be quite elderly and may not tolerate multiple laser excisions especially as it is not certain they will get a malignancy and surgery does not guarantee that they will not.

Erythroplakia, or red patch, is a less common but sinister potentially malignant lesion; it is often mixed with white speckles or areas. Sub-mucous fibrosis occurs predominantly in Asians and is caused by chewing the areca nut. It is very common worldwide but not necessarily within the UK. Patients will experience burning of the mucosa and sensitivity to spicy foods. The mucosa has a blanched appearance and an increased risk of malignant transformation. Fibrous bands form beneath the mucosa leading to progressive decrease in mouth opening. Sub-mucous fibrosis is very challenging for the clinician, not only attempting to help with the progressive trismus but monitoring the oral mucosa for malignant change when mouth opening is inadequate.

In conclusion the management of potentially malignant conditions of the oral mucosa is awkward because they may be mimicked by many lesions without malignant potential. They are often not homogenous; most of them do not become malignant and there is no universally agreed management strategy. Management of each lesion must be dictated by an experienced clinician and not delegated to trainees.

In our experience most mistakes in management we have seen have been related to lesions on the lateral border of the tongue which were not taken seriously enough. An apparently small area of mucosal damage caused by dental trauma can be mimicked by invasive cancer. Dental trauma must be observed to heal completely (not just improved) after removal of the apparent cause before a patient may be reassured and discharged from follow up. A small tongue cancer

Field change. The patient has widespread dysplasia around the mouth which produced multiple metachronous tumours. Very difficult to deal with. The sutures are from a recent biopsy.

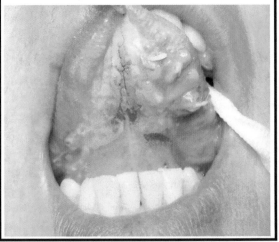

54. <u>Introduction to Salivary Gland Swellings</u>

You should expect to see a good number of swellings of the salivary glands in any OMFS department. These will mostly be caused by obstruction to the outflow of saliva from the glands and less commonly due to tumours, most of which will be benign.

Most common are mucoceles in the lower lip. Mucoceles are pseudocysts (no lining) that consist of saliva which has extravasated into the surrounding soft tissues usually consequent upon damage to the salivary gland ducts, in this case by the teeth. Their treatment is removal of the gland which feeds the swelling. The procedure requires exposing the small mucous glands via a vertical incision within the oral mucosa. There are multiple small nerves ascending to the vermillion of the lower lip which can be damaged during the procedure, leading to numbness. It is easy to miss removing the precise small gland causing the swelling so this is a procedure that should always be carried out by someone who has been trained to do it.

A ranula is a mucocele of the sublingual salivary gland. This is usually seen as a soft swelling in the floor of the mouth; sometimes the swelling may penetrate below the mylohyoid muscle into the neck and be seen as a soft swelling in the submandibular area. This is called a plunging ranula but the mechanism and treatment are the same.

The definitive treatment of a ranula is removal of the sublingual gland but access is difficult so that a general anaesthetic is nearly always indicated. The sublingual gland is shaped like a tadpole with the thinner end forming into the duct which is closely associated with the deep part of the submandibular gland. It does not normally shell out easily; it is more like a controlled tearing and there is risk of damage to the lingual nerve and duct of the submandibular gland.

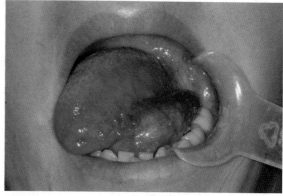

Ranula

Furthermore there is a healthy network of vessels in the floor of the mouth which can result in prolonged bleeding. Removal of the roof of the ranula under local anaesthetic will relieve the symptoms in the short term but it is likely to recur. However in children the chances of recurrence are much less and this may often be used as a definitive treatment.

Strictures or, more commonly, stones in the ducts of the submandibular glands can cause swelling associated with eating. The resulting salivary stasis can lead to painful ascending infection - sialadentis. The submandibular gland is more frequently involved than the parotid. Removal of a stone which is causing obstruction from the duct in the floor of the mouth may be relatively straightforward under local anaesthetic if it is located anteriorly. This can produce immediate relief of symptoms but there may be other stones in the gland which may cause problems in the future. These may sometimes show up on plain radiographs but are better demonstrated by an ultrasound scan. After removal of a stone from the duct the wound should be left open and the patient

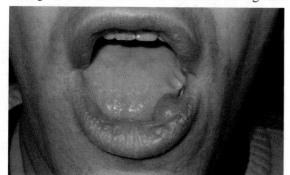

A typical mucocoele in the lip

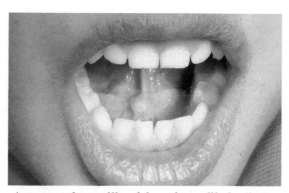

A stone at the papilla of the submandibular duct

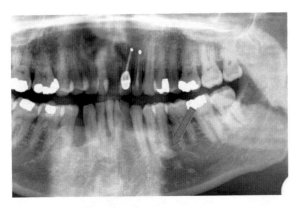

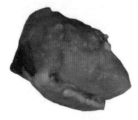

Some stones may be seen on X-ray as in this OPG above, otherwise ultrasound imaging is most reliable. Below the stone after removal.

encouraged to stimulate saliva to decrease the likelihood of stricture formation in the duct.

A submandibular gland which has experienced obstruction and recurrent sialadentis over a prolonged period will probably need its removal to prevent further symptoms. Patients who get immediate relief from removal of a stone from the floor of the mouth should be warned that such surgery may be needed at some time in the future.

Obstruction of the outflow of the parotid gland may be due to a stricture more commonly than a stone. This may be demonstrated with sialography where a radiopaque contrast is injected into the duct to enable an image of the ductal system to be made. This may be therapeutic as well as diagnostic as it may flush out plugs of mucous which are causing obstruction.

Less frequently a stone may be formed in the parotid gland and cause obstruction in the duct by coming to rest at the papilla. Incising the papilla over the stone may produce scarring leading to a stricture later. This risk may be minimized by making a C-shaped incision over the stone behind the papilla to remove the stone and to leave it open to drain. A stone which is mobile rather than stuck may be removed by basket retrieval. A very thin wire is passed into the duct of the gland, a plunger is pressed and the basket opens

up and is withdrawn, pulling the stone with it. This may be used concurrently with a sialo-endoscope which enables the inside of the duct to be visualized; it has the advantage of not using radiation. Sometimes strictures of the parotid may be relieved (as least temporarily) by dilation with an arterial balloon catheter.

Salivary gland tumours are most common in the parotid gland. Pleomorphic adenoma is the commonest; although benign it can increase in size very slowly over a number of years and spread beyond the capsule of the gland and therefore need to be removed with a margin of normal tissue as with a malignant tumour. If not completely removed with a margin they have a propensity to recur several years later and seed in several different parts of the face and become very difficult to control in the long term. They can also give rise to a malignant tumour from the benign tissue. The typical operation for removal of pleomorphic adenoma is removal of all of the superficial parotid gland i.e. all of the gland superficial to the facial nerve which is about 80% of the total volume of the gland. Tumours arising in the 20% deep part of the gland are very rare.

Warthin's tumours are the next most common, also benign. It is not essential to remove them but if they are visible on the face they may be removed for cosmesis. Warthin's can be bilateral and can sometimes cause pain which would be an indication for removal; they most frequently affect women and are associated with smoking.

Tumours of the submandibular gland and sublingual glands are much less common than of the parotid but when they do occur are more likely to be malignant. There are several different types of malignant salivary gland tumours but the least uncommon are mucoepidermoid, adenocystic and adenocarcinoma. Mucoepidermoid carcinomas come in different grades of malignancy; some behave fairly innocuously, being more like benign tumours with the higher grade ones behaving like a squamous cancer. Adenocystic carcinomas are malignant but tend to grow very slowly and have a propensity to grow along nerves. They have a very good 5 year survival rate but tend to recur many years later while adenocarcinomas behave as classical malignant tumours.

The operation you are most likely to see for salivary tumours is superficial parotidectomy. The parotid gland superficial to the facial nerve where most of the tumours originate is removed usually through an incision just anterior to the pinna of the ear. The facial nerve is identified as it leaves the stylomastoid foramen

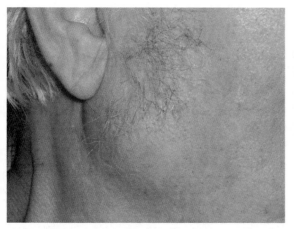

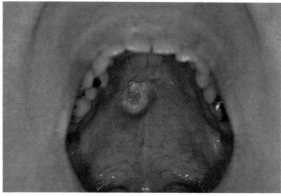

Occasionally tumours may arise in minor salivary glands. This is a pleomorphic adenoma.

A parotid lump. Most likely a pleomorphic adenoma in the superficial part of the gland. Examination should include checking the external ear and side of head for skin cancer least this be metastatic cancer in intra-parotid lymph nodes and facial nerve function which will always be normal with benign tumour. The suspected diagnosis should be confirmed by fine needle aspiration cytology and an ultrasound scan or CT will demonstrate the extent of the tumour.

secretomotor fibres from the gland stimulate sweat glands in the skin. Patients should be warned before surgery.

Removal of the submandibular gland is a fairly straightforward operation approached through a skin crease below the mandible to give the best cosmesis. The incision should be low enough to avoid the mandibular branch of the facial nerve. The gland is normally shelled out quite easily unless there has been prolonged sialadentis causing fibrosis; the duct of the gland is tied before being cut. The lingual nerve which crosses the duct should be observed and preserved. Access to the sublingual gland is from the floor of the mouth but its removal is awkward as it does not shell out easily and the submandibular gland duct and lingual nerve can potentially be damaged.

Imaging for swellings is primarily by ultrasound. This will tell the clinician whether the swelling is multifocal, bilateral, the size and whether it originates in the salivary tissue or in the lymph glands within the parotid gland which may be enlarged by metastatic squamous cancer from the skin.

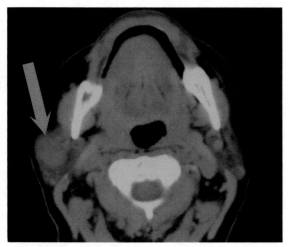

A parotid is defined in the superficial parotid by computerised tomography (CT)

and followed forward leaving it intact but removing the gland superficial to it. Afterwards the patient can expect temporary facial nerve weakness because the nerve has been manipulated but this can be expected to recover, assuming the nerve has not been cut. Permanent facial nerve paralysis is very deforming; the affected side of the face will droop which will be progressive as tone is lost from the facial muscles. Many patients will exhibit Frey's syndrome (gustatory sweating) after parotidectomy. They will experience sweating on the side of the face as

55. <u>Keeping out of Trouble</u>

Performing well in your new job should be fairly easy. All that the Consultants will probably expect is for their new trainee to be conscientious, enthusiastic and to learn. Avoiding trouble should be easy but nevertheless this can occur. Here we have listed the best things not to do; it is based on our observations of many years of hospital practice, tales of woe we have heard in the form of gossip from colleagues and monitoring the GDC and GMC websites. Be aware that many formal disciplinary issues are started because of complaints promoted by personal animosity from colleagues so do try not to fall out with anyone.

We advise that it is prudent to come to work dressed in a professional manner. This does not mean dressing formally (you will have to see patients without a necktie or sleeves) but tidily. In particular everyone should have clean shoes and gentlemen should be clean shaven or if they have facial hair it should be neat and not stubble because they couldn't be bothered to shave. Ladies should not wear short party dresses and high heels if they want to be taken seriously by patients and colleagues. We advise you not to:-

1. Make inaccurate travel claims. Always make a contemporaneous record when you travel as part of your job to ensure your mileage claims are accurate. If anyone is out to get you this is the first thing they will check on.

2. Use the hospital internet to look at pornographic web sites even if it is in hospital residential accommodation. Their use is always monitored and people have been sacked or reported to the General Dental Council for it, so they will not be able to make an exception for you.

3. Make changes in the medical management of a patient on the wards on your own initiative. You should always report medical problems or complications to someone more senior who should be a medically qualified doctor.

4. Prescribe medication for yourself, your family or any member of the hospital staff .

5. Treat family or friends or anyone outside of the normal referral mechanism. If a member of staff asks you to treat their dental pain ask the Consultant what the policy is before you do so and always make sure that they are registered on the hospital patient administration system and that hospital notes are written.

6. Give opinions on diagnosis and management of patients outside the framework of guidance given to you by your Consultants.

7. Make any form of sexual advance to anyone while at work.

8. Refuse to see any patients that you have been requested to without getting senior advice or guidance.

9. Keep quiet about complications you have caused or errors you have made. It will become apparent at a later date and then you will appear untrustworthy. Always come clean to the Consultant and explain what has happened and the circumstances. Remember everyone has made mistakes and misjudgements and the Consultant will be older than you and have therefore made more. However, we have to confess it difficult to take anyone seriously who has taken out a wrong tooth.

10. Regularly turn up late.

11. Be overconfident in your abilities, experience or judgement. Always ask advice when not exactly sure and never allow anyone, be they patient or staff, to think that you are more senior or experienced than you are.

12. Allow anyone to think you are a doctor rather than dental surgeon.

11. Tell lies.

12. Fabricate data for any research or audit project you are involved with.

13. Make inaccurate or misleading claims on job applications

14. Consult medical records, be they written notes, X-rays or pathology reports for friends, relatives or colleagues where you have no legitimate professional duty to do so.

15. Take photographs of patients on mobile phones or other personal devices. Show photographs of any patients outside of a clinical setting or store images of patients on your own equipment. If you are involved with taking patient images read the hospital's image policy (probably on their intranet).

16. Be rude to anyone, either staff or patient whatever the provocation.

17. Slag anyone off on social media.

56. <u>Dedication</u>

This book is dedicated to the generations of young dental surgeons who have passed through our departments over the years and who have inspired us with their energy, enthusiasm, and thirst for knowledge and practical experience. By so doing they have enriched our professional lives. And in particular those who have left behind a legacy of clearly legible, concise and dated clinical notes. Not like this:

(Locum SHO Lincoln December 2003)

And also to all those who have attended our lectures and courses and have given us constructive criticism and feedback which has steered us on the path to improvement. And not like this:

(Dentist on the Ward course Lincoln 2005)

57. <u>Feedback</u>

This book is an ongoing project with a new edition updated each year with additional chapters. It is our intention to add more chapters with concise essential medical and surgical information for patient management and non-specialist dentistry examinations.

We would be grateful for feedback to know what parts should be omitted, which topics should be added and anything which you believe to be inaccurate or out of date.

Please tick the Chapters which you found interesting or useful and put a cross next to those which were not helpful. Please scan and email your response to DOW@sorejaw.co.uk or post to DOW 21 Chestnut Street, Lincoln LN13HB. If you don't want to deface your book the form can be downloaded from www.dentist-on-the-ward.co.uk.

Thank you. *Andrew and Leo*

1. Why work in Oral and Maxillofacial Surgery?
2. Applying for a job in Oral and Maxillofacial Surgery
3. Getting the best from your student attachment or elective
4. Education, Personal Development and Appraisal
5. Information, Data Protection and Confidentiality
6. Pre-employment Health Assessment and the Blood Borne Viruses
7. Hospital Cross Infection Control: MRSA, Clostridium Difficile and Hand Hygiene
8. Inoculation (needlestick) Injuries
9. Day Surgery
10. The Ward: its Staff and Routines
11. Preparation for Theatre
12. Consent for Hospital Treatment
13. Working in the Operating Theatre
14. Scrubbing and Gowning
15. Routine Post-Operative Care
16. Post-Operative Complications
17. Understanding the Intensive Care Unit
18. Being On Call, Accidents and Emergencies

19. Wound Closure - Skin Suturing
20. Dealing with Bleeding from the Mouth
21. Examination of the Injured Face
22. Imaging for Facial Fractures
23. Admitting a Patient with a Facial Fracture
24. Admitting a Patient with a Dental Abscess

25. You Should Know About Retrobulbar Haemorrhage
26. Medical Emergencies
27. Resuscitation
28. Examination of Cardiovascular and Respiratory Systems
29. The Sterile Supply Service
30. Surgical Instruments
31. Minor Oral Surgery
32. The Management of Impacted Teeth
33. Histopathology
34. Venepuncture - Taking a Blood Sample
35. Venepuncture - Inserting a Venflon IV Cannula
36. Blood Tests: Ordering and Interpretation
37. Blood Tests - Haematology
38. Blood Tests - Biochemistry
39. Blood Tests - Immunology
40. Understanding Fluid and Blood Replacement
41. Prescribing Medication in the Hospital
42. Understanding the Anaesthetist
43. Understanding Tracheostomy
44. The Head & Neck Cancer Multidisciplinary Team (MDT)
45. Understanding a Major Cancer Case
46. Understanding Radiotherapy and its Oral Complications
47. Understanding Chemotherapy and its Oral Complications
48. Understanding Diabetes and its Impact on Surgery
49. Medication Related Osteonecrosis of the Jaws
50. Anticoagulation and Surgery
51. Understanding Orthognathic Surgery
52. Introduction to Facial Skin Cancer
53. Understanding Potentially Malignant Oral Disorders
54. Introduction to Salivary Gland Swellings
55. Keeping out of Trouble

Additional comments. In particular corrections or anything you recommend to be included in future editions. Thank you

DOW@sorejaw.co.uk   DOW 21 Chestnut Street, Lincoln. LN1 3HB

187

53724202R00109

Made in the USA
Charleston, SC
18 March 2016